D0729524

"Lori Hope writes with an eloquence and authenticity th[...] readers. She expertly takes cancer caregivers and surviv[...] helps us strengthen ourselves and revive the precious g[...] us do so even in the face of cancer's many blurts and blunders. If you or a loved one have been touched by cancer, *Help Me Live* is required reading."

—Greg Anderson, author of *Cancer: 50 Essential Things to Do*, Founder and CEO,
  Cancer Recovery Foundation Group

"Even though I am a twenty-year survivor, I needed to be reminded about what people in the throes of cancer need, and Lori Hope's book is perfect."

—Kathy La Tour, Editor-at-Large, *Cure* magazine

"It's a wonderful work that both eloquently and simply reminds us that empathy, humanity, respect, and dignity for each other should never fall victim to cancer. In working over fifteen years as an oncology social worker, it seemed as if Lori Hope had been sitting alongside me catching the rich insights and poignant narratives of our clients and then beautifully crafted *Help Me Live* to assist the world in truly understanding how one best helps the cancer patient."

—Win Boerckel, LCSW, MSW, Director of Social Service, CancerCare of Long Island

"Lori Hope's masterful storytelling and clear explanations are invaluable for cancer survivors, helping you understand (and forgive) others' hurtful words and actions, and encouraging you to direct family and friends to responses that help. This book is a gift for caregivers and everyone who knows someone who is going though illness."

—Wendy Harpham, MD, author of *Happiness in a Storm*, *Diagnosis: Cancer*, and
  Only 10 Seconds to Care: Help and Hope for Busy Clinicians

"Lori Hope, who has been through it all, both as a cancer patient and a loving supporter of other cancer patients, offers guidance that is always sensitive and often deeply illuminating. Please, please, read this book!"

—Barbara Ehrenreich, author of *Bright–Sided: How Positive Thinking Is Undermining America* and *Nickel and Dimed*

"*Help Me Live* is beautifully written and offers extraordinary pearls of wisdom on love, on hope, on survivorship, on friendship—in the face of a cancer diagnosis. As a survivor herself she takes us on heartfelt journey—and we are stronger and more courageous because of it."

—Laurie Fenton Ambrose, President and CEO, Lung Cancer Alliance

"Drawing on her experience, those of many others, and that of a number of leading health professionals, Lori provides sensible and sensitive guidelines for helping those with cancer and their families to live better. If you or a loved one is struggling with cancer, don't be without Hope."

—David Spiegel, MD, Stanford University, author of *Living Beyond Limits*

"*Help Me Live* is a deeply moving exploration of the complex range of emotions that arise in the face of illness. Both patients and caregivers can enter their roles with greater acceptance and love from reading the experiences and interviews by Lori Hope."

—Susan Halpern, MSW, author of *The Etiquette of Illness*

"Patients with cancer often say to me, 'It's bad enough to have cancer, but would you BELIEVE what someone said to me the other day?' Those expressions are not easily forgotten, when they caused either pain or joy. I really like Lori's use of these common expressions as the base for suggesting good etiquette and kind manners in talking to someone who has a serious illness."

—Jimmie Holland, MD, Memorial Sloan-Kettering Cancer Center,
  author of *The Human Side of Cancer*

"The advice, comments, and suggestions contained within *Help Me Live* are valuable to cancer patients, their families, friends, caregivers, physicians, and therapists as well as any compassionate individual."

—Jo Ellen Lezotte, past President, The Caner League, Inc.

"This is a book every cancer survivor, as well as those who share our world, need to read. She says the words that none of us wants to say out loud and offers realistic explanations of how we all need to relate to our disease. This book can offer a great deal of comfort to those starting on the path of living with cancer."

—Kathryn Joosten, actress, *The West Wing*, *Desperate Housewives*, and *Scrubs*

"As a two-time survivor of breast cancer and a journalist, I found *Help Me Live* to be informative, touching, and even funny—and when it comes to cancer, you need a sense of humor. The author certainly lives up to her name."

—Laura Marquez, ABC News correspondent

"Always compassionate and pragmatic, Lori gives voice to other survivors who candidly share their insights and experiences. *Help Me Live* breaks new ground with sections on children and young adults and cultural considerations—truly a wonderful resource for all of us."

—Peggy McGuire, Executive Director, Women's Cancer Resource Center

"As an oncology nurse with over fourteen years of experience I have learned many truths by listening to my clients. When I read Lori's book, I found myself nodding in recognition of many of these truths. She writes exquisitely of the emotions and the roller-coaster ride of a cancer diagnosis and treatment. As a nurse educator, I plan to share this book with my students to try and give them some insight into the common experiences that many cancer patients have, as well as the uncommon ones."

—Patricia Reilly, California State University School of Nursing

"This book is a gift to anyone who has been touched by cancer—and that is most of us. At the core of *Help Me Live* Lori Hope offers a succinct and strong message—JUST BE THERE. In those three words she offers guidance, strength, and hope and underscores the importance of sharing our stories."

—Nancy L. Snyderman, M.D., F.A.C.S., NBC News Chief Medical Editor,
  Associate Professor Head and Neck Surgery, University of Pennsylvania

"Here's the twenty-first thing you should know: This book is invaluable for anyone diagnosed with cancer and for anyone who has a family member or friend battling the disease. Lori Hope, a lung cancer survivor, writes intimately, poignantly, poetically, and humorously as she tells it like it is."

—Marc Silver, author of *Breast Cancer Husband: Help Your Wife (and Yourself) during Diagnosis, Treatment, and Beyond*

"As someone who works every day with lung cancer patients, I know the deep wounds that careless words—including the question, 'Did you smoke?'—can inflict. Lori Hope shows you how to do the opposite, how to help someone with cancer heal by taking away the blame and stigma. Read this book, cover to cover, and help someone live. I did."

—Sheila von Driska, Executive Director, Bonnie J. Addario Lung Cancer Foundation

"While many books are available to guide people with cancer and their families through the physical and emotional upheaval of their journey, few are dedicated to how to help—and avoid hurting—others with our words. In *Help Me Live*, Lori Hope has created a masterpiece of compelling and heartfelt words of healing that should be required reading for doctors, family, and friends of anyone traversing the cancer landscape."

—Regina Vidaver, PhD, Executive Director, The National Lung Cancer Partnership

"Lori Hope's refreshingly candid voice cuts a gentle, steady path through confusion and discomfort. She's a true expert in her field."

—Hope Edelman, author of *Motherless Daughters*

"*Help Me Live* is personal, practical, and heartfelt and makes it easier to navigate the gritty realities of what to say and do if you want to help."

—Jean Shinoda Bolen, MD, author of *Close to the Bone: Life-Threatening Illness and the Search for Meaning*

"Lori's book is filled with warmth, practical advice, and perspectives that can help start a great conversation with those we care about who are affected by cancer . . . [moving] us from feeling fear or hesitation to connection and community when we need it most. Definitely worth reading!"

—Margaret Stauffer, Program Director, Cancer Support Community, San Francisco Bay Area

"In her new chapter on gender issues, Lori looks at the differences between men and women in the face of major illness. From my own experience, it was so familiar to read about the female need to have a mate who most of the time only needs to listen, versus the male tendency to rush to fix what ever he perceives is wrong."

—Richard Anderson, past President, Well Spouse™ Association

help me live

---

20 things
people with cancer
want you to know

revised and expanded

Lori Hope

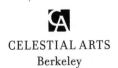

CELESTIAL ARTS
Berkeley

Published in the United States by Celestial Arts, an imprint of the
Crown Publishing Group, a division of Random House, Inc., New York.
www.crownpublishing.com
www.tenspeed.com

Celestial Arts and the Celestial Arts colophon are registered trademarks
of Random House, Inc.

Grateful acknowledgment is made to the *Journal of Transpersonal Psychology* for
permission to reprint an excerpt from "On Being a Support Person" by Ken Wilbur,
copyright © 1988. Reprinted by permission of Daniel L. Gaylinn, Executive Director,
Association of Transpersonal Psychology, and the author.

Library of Congress Cataloging-in-Publication Data
Hope, Lori.
 Help me live : 20 things people with cancer want you to know /
Lori Hope. — Rev. ed.
      p. cm.
 Includes bibliographical references and index.
 1. Cancer—Popular works. 2. Cancer—Psychological aspects.
I.Title.
 RC263.H67 2011
 616.99'4—dc23
                          2011015572

ISBN 978-1-58761-149-0 (pbk.)

Printed in the United States

Design by Nancy Austin and Chloe Rawlins

10 9 8 7 6 5 4 3 2 1

This book is dedicated to

Norman Crasilneck,
October 6, 1926–June 28, 2010,

forever my father and one of the brightest stars in my universe,
whose inspiriting sunniness, generosity, and disarming sense
of humor hearten me every single day.

Help Me Live *is given in love to David.*

Contents

Part II: A Quick Guide to Cancerquette

foreword
by Rachel Naomi Remen, MD

THIS IS NOT A BOOK ABOUT CANCER, it is a book about you. About the importance of your love. About the many helpful ways of being there for someone else. About never having to worry about not being enough again.

There are times when our hearts simply do not have the right words and we feel that we are not enough. But if you worry about saying the right thing to someone with cancer, you already are just what is needed, someone who wants to help at a hard time, someone to whom it matters. In *Help Me Live*, Lori Hope offers us the right words. If you are reading this book, you already have the right heart.

I have had Crohn's disease for fifty-eight years. In thinking back on my own experience with dark times and life-altering illness, not as a doctor but as a patient, the things I remember that were most helpful were not expert advice. They were small things, things that connected me to normal people, to normal life, to the future. The people who did this for me did so in many different ways—all of them were heartfelt. There was the friend who traveled two hours to see me and found me so self-absorbed that I continued reading my book and ignored her presence in the room. "HOW RUDE YOU ARE!" she exclaimed and burst into tears.

My surgery had left made me feeling hopelessly different. It was as if a thick plate of glass had fallen between me and all the people who were whole. With just four words, she had shattered it and reconnected me to them. I could hear them and touch them. I might have lost part of my body but I was still a card-carrying part member of the human race, an equal who had the power to hurt others and also to love them. For a moment I was shocked and then I remember thinking "I am not an invalid. She would never have talked to an invalid like that." My sense of brokenness simply vanished and for the first time in weeks, I began to laugh.

Then there was my surgeon who visited me in the hospital the day before my first twelve-hour abdominal surgery. He handed me an envelope and in it was a signed pass to leave the surgical ward for a few hours. Seeing my puzzled look, he suggested that I might want to go out and have a manicure. A while back he had asked his wife and daughters how he might be of help to his female patients the day before their surgery, and they had suggested he offer this opportunity. Tears filled my eyes. Outwardly I had looked calm, while but in reality I had been terrified of dying on the operating table the next day. But no one suggests a manicure to someone they believe will die the next day. Getting a manicure meant I had a future.

I have come to believe that when we speak and act from the heart we are all healers. So the trick is not to become someone different . . . but to become more confident in expressing the caring person you already are. That sort of confidence comes only from life experience. Lori Hope has taken the time to ask real questions and listen deeply to hundreds of real people with cancer. To write their stories down so that we can have the chance to listen to them too. To learn from them.

Help Me Live is about a great many things you may not have known about having cancer and a great many things you may not have known about yourself. It is a book about finding the courage to speak and act from the heart when times are tough.

Ultimately, *Help Me Live* is a book of personal discovery. Somewhere within its pages you will come to believe in yourself and the power of your caring to make a difference, to strengthen the will to live in another person and help them to heal. Once we have confidence, we can each do this in ways as unique as our fingerprints. Without Lori's book, we might not have known how much we matter and found the courage to do something about it.

Rachel Naomi Remen, MD, author of *Kitchen Table Wisdom: Stories That Heal*, and *My Grandfather's Blessings: Stories of Strength, Refuge, and Belonging*

preface to the revised edition

We shall not cease from exploration
And the end of all our exploring
Will be to arrive where we started
And know the place for the first time.

—T. S. Eliot, from *The Four Quartets*

I THOUGHT I UNDERSTOOD CANCER.

As a medical reporter, documentary producer, and caregiver, I had seen it from myriad sides. Having interviewed dozens of doctors and scientists and read reams about the scourge that will strike one in three women and half of all men during their lifetime, I thought I knew plenty.

In the process of making two films about right-to-die issues, I had metaphorically stepped into the shoes of cancer patients whose lives I chronicled, gazing into eyes fearful, peaceful, or tear-filled, and listening to strikingly different tales of hope and healing. I navigated the sand-shifting terrain of cancer alongside friends and family. After my cousin Barbara emerged glassy-eyed from her breast biopsy and mouthed flatly, "I have cancer," I helped steady her through the hurricane of medical appointments that followed; when my dear friend, Missy, fought colon cancer at age forty-three, I ferreted out information about conventional treatments, clinical trials, and complementary therapies, crossing the Mexican border with her to tour eerily hushed, glossy-floored adobe clinics. And when my best childhood friend and cousin, Billee, underwent a bone marrow transplant to rid her body of cancer, we shared quiet hope in her darkened hospital room.

Indeed, I thought I knew cancer. But in 2002, when I was diagnosed myself, everything I thought I understood evanesced. The magic carpet of privilege I did not realize I had ridden throughout my life abruptly stopped, and I found myself free falling, not knowing when, where, or how I would land. That proverbial fall from innocence began during a routine checkup, when my doctor felt a hardening in my abdomen.

"It's probably nothing," Dr. Aye said, "but with your history, we should check it out." I had a uterine fibroid tumor and feared it had grown. Though a CT scan revealed my abdomen was clear—oh, how my husband and I celebrated after the halo-headed radiologist held my hand and told me I had impacted stool (read: constipation)—I received a call from Dr. Aye two hours later.

"The radiologist took another look at your scan, and saw something on your lung."

I had lung cancer.

Even though over the past two decades I had seen firsthand many inspiring tales of survival—even though I knew diagnosis did not equal death—I had never heard of a lung cancer *survivor*. Terror-struck, I desperately needed support. And hope. Although my community speedily rallied with love, compassion, and generous intentions, a few unwittingly said or did things that did not comfort.

"You'll be okay if you just think positively." *If I can't, does that mean I'll make my tumor grow?*

"Did you smoke?" *Yes, but I quit almost twenty years ago. So do you think I deserve it?*

"I'm so sorry. My great aunt just died of cancer." *Is that what I have to look forward to?*

Some of my health-care providers suffered foot-in-mouth disease, too. "Although your tumor is very small," said my oncologist, "and we don't see others on the CT scan, they could open you up on the operating table and find hundreds of tumors too small to be detected by the scan." When I heard those words, terror shot through my psyche like poison. I could only hope the cancer had not spread like that through my body!

2 2 2

I realized that although I knew a lot about the disease, I did not know as much as I thought about its ravages on the psyche. Talking with others in my post-cancer-treatment support group, I discovered that my experiences were far too common. Though my "Cancer Club" pals and I laughed about the often-hilarious faux pas that others and even *we* had committed—after all, who *hasn't* blurted words they wish they could recant?—our pain cut deep, and we bemoaned the fear, shock, or compassion that precluded our sharing information about what would really help not just us, but cancer combatants to follow. That's why I decided to undertake a project to let other voices speak for hope-hungry survivors too stunned, vulnerable, or considerate to speak for themselves. (Note: Throughout this book, anyone living with a cancer diagnosis is referred to as a survivor.)

During 2003 and 2004, I interviewed survivors of diverse ages, backgrounds, and diagnoses; experts in psychology, social work, communications, and conventional and mind-body medicine; and surveyed scores of cancer survivors to write the first edition of *Help Me Live: 20 Things People with Cancer Want You to Know.*

〜〜〜

After the book launched in 2005, I heard from not only cancer caregivers and survivors, but also from individuals who thought a "20 Things" book should be written about their various conditions. This reinforced to me the clearly universal nature of the principles illustrated and espoused in *Help Me Live*, which apply not just to people with cancer, but anyone with diseases and conditions from multiple sclerosis to posttraumatic stress disorder. This recently became more apparent when a *New York Times* blog post, "When Friends Disappear During a Health Crisis," inspired more than two hundred comments.

More important, in the ensuing years I found that, even though I knew far more than "plenty," there was much more to learn, explore, and share, partly because the world had grown in ever-broadening dimensions.

Between 2002, when I was diagnosed, and 2011, the Internet exploded from a superhighway to an infinite universe with space stations in the millions. Online communities providing anonymous, 24/7 support mushroomed, and the virtual world—a petri dish for the young adult cancer community—burgeoned, along with social networking, video, and cancer support sites, and the blogosphere. At the same time, hopeful new cancer treatments emerged, and the American Cancer Society reported that 67 percent of those diagnosed with cancer would survive for at least five years.

Another change in the Cancersphere came in 2008, when the National Institute of Medicine (NIM) issued a report saying that quality cancer care must integrate the psychosocial domain (emotional and social problems caused by the disease). As psychiatrist Jimmie Holland, MD, founding president of the American Psychosocial and Behavioral Oncology Society and author of *The Human Side of Cancer*, told me, "It's a blockbuster for us [The Alliance for Quality Psychosocial Cancer Care] because we've never had public policy support before like that. The National Institute of Medicine put out a book called *Care for the Whole Patient*. . . . now used widely all over the world."

The report and book have helped destigmatize and normalize cancer, as have two recent television series whose protagonists have cancer: *The Big C*, starring Laura Linney, and *Breaking Bad*, starring Bryan Cranston, who portrays a lung cancer patient who's never smoked. Many journalists have also spotlighted the subject. *Time* magazine, *NBC Today*, and other prominent media have trumpeted words and actions that help, hurt, or heal. A blog of that name, *what helps. what hurts. what heals.*, reached a worldwide audience after CarePages.com, which provides free websites for ill people, invited me to write a weekly column. That led to more exploration and feedback, and the continued reinforcement of overarching principles of communication that apply not only to people with cancer but to anyone facing serious life challenges.

⊒⊒⊒

As much as the world changed between 2005 and 2011, in some respects it stayed stubbornly the same. Foot-in-mouth disease remained as virulent as the common cold. And even though the stigma of cancer diminished somewhat, ignorance and insensitivity continued to add proverbial insult to the profound injury of cancer. As life—or our passage through it—accelerated to warp speed, many of us found it more difficult to hold our tongues before blurting something we wish we hadn't, or to even take a moment to consider our loved ones' needs.

Clearly, with all that had changed and stayed the same, it was time to revise *Help Me Live*. It would not only expand on more popular subjects such as cancer and gender, young adult cancer, and positive psychology, but would also revisit what survivors want people without cancer to know. Hence a new survey that reached more than six hundred survivors from ages eighteen to eighty-eight across the globe, from Alaska to Australia, asking what words and actions are most appreciated and reviled.

It was also time to address not just how friends and loved ones can best support survivors, but how survivors can best support themselves. Although *Help Me Live* was not intended for them, survivors read the book to find validation, comfort, hope, and a sense of community in others' stories. I realized that I had not just an opportunity but also an obligation to foster that hope. Thus, you will find tips about how to keep hope alive when external forces such as news headlines or gaffes threaten to dent, dash, or destroy it. This, plus new survivor stories and intimate lessons from my own unexpected challenges await you. You will also find a new, expanded Cancerquette guide for busy caregivers, friends, and loved ones with just enough time for bullet points, lists, and concrete suggestions.

Whether you are reading this because someone you care about has cancer or another serious illness, or you're a survivor attempting to understand and forgive someone whose words or actions have wounded you, I hope this book will convince you that anyone can develop the skills to do what they want more than anything: to help those they care about through life's harshest challenges, and help them live. Numerous studies show that social support increases wellness and longevity in healthy individuals. Whether or not it does the same for cancer survivors, love and compassion indisputably enhance the quality of everyone's life, including the supporter's.

May you find understanding, encouragement, self-forgiveness, self-compassion, peace, and support in the pages that follow. Giving support may be as simple as just being there. As psychiatrist David Spiegel, Director of Stanford University's Center on Stress and Health said of physicians, "We're trained to treat crying as bleeding, to apply direct pressure to stop it." But in the case of emotions, that may not be appropriate. When training support group leaders, Dr. Spiegel advises, "If you see somebody crying, don't just do something—stand there."

Thank you for standing here with all of us who have been impacted by cancer and for reading this revised and expanded edition of *Help Me Live: 20 Things People with Cancer Want You to Know*. To quote a new statement that people with cancer want others to know, a statement that I could not help but add, "I am more grateful than I can say for your care, compassion, and support."

Thank you for helping us live.

introduction

What do we live for, if it is not to make life less difficult for each other?

—George Eliot

I AWAKEN IN MY DORMITORY-SIZE room and can hardly wait to peek outside at the young, thin-limbed maple tree silhouetted against the 6 a.m. lilac-gray sky. What a thrill to be on my own, poised to finish the final chapter of this book, a book about cancer. No, a book about hope—about listening—about being there.

On a private writing retreat at a wooded monastery in northwest Washington, named for St. Placid, a monk rescued from drowning by a fellow monk, I feel happier than I can remember. Having survived cancer, I just returned from Cancer as a Turning Point, a free conference that freshened my heart with hope. My nineteen-year-old son, Brett, recently called my cell phone to ask if I know anyone who needs a newspaper subscription which he wants to purchase out of compassion for the salesman outside Safeway. And, finally, my husband left a voicemail saying with love rich as fudge, "I miss you so much." It doesn't get much better than this.

As I move through the hallway in my slippers, I step gingerly to avoid disturbing the other retreatants sleeping behind doors labeled for Benedictines such as Heloise and Hrotsvit of Gandersheim. In the fluorescent-lit communal kitchen that still smells of popcorn from the night before, I turn a stainless steel knob next to the faucet, pumping 190-degree water into a plastic cone to brew my go-juice, and leave the kitchen, quietly shutting the door behind me.

Laptop cradled tightly against my left ribs—ribs split apart two years ago so a lobe of my lung could be removed—I walk through the propped-open door labeled, "Parlor," eight feet across the hall from Hadewijch, named for the Benedictine who coined "Love conquers all things." I gently place my computer on the loveseat and bend to lift the brass doorstop. I close the door so I can rustle papers, tap the keyboard, and talk to myself without disturbing the man in Hadewijch, an egg-shaped man with silver eyebrows and plaid shirt, a Leprechaun-lumberjack hybrid who told me the night before that he recently lost his wife of fifty years. Five decades. Can you imagine?

Safe in the well-insulated parlor, my fingers type with impunity. Deep in thought, calm and focused, a loud KAPLUNK! shoots my pulse from 60 to 100. The door, which I had closed so gently, had apparently not closed completely. Natural law had asserted its rule to complete the action.

If it had been able to speak, this is what the heavy hunk of wood might have declared: "The road to hell is paved with the best intentions. Due to circumstances both within and beyond your control, you have and may continue to unintentionally disturb people you wish to avoid hurting at all cost."

I relax into a quiet laugh and ask myself, "So what is the point of writing a book about supporting people with cancer, since you will likely hurt them anyway—since they may hear words differently than you intended them, or attach a different or distorted meaning to your actions?"

The Point

In deciding how to act or what to say to the ill, infirm, or suffering, we rely on advice or examples presented by role models from childhood on. Real-life people and events, fairy tales and stories, entertainment, and popular and news media show us what works and fails, teaching right from wrong. The problem is, we do not live in a world of immutable right and wrong, black and white; rather, we make our way through a spectral universe broader and richer than most of us have the capacity, imagination, or patience to visualize. Age, diagnosis, prognosis, gender, and cultural background help determine reactions. What comforts one may crush another. Each person's psyche is as unique as her fingerprints.

In addition, people differ not only from one another, but within themselves, depending on the day—especially days made significant by doctors' appointments, anniversaries or special occasions—or even time of day. Plus, cancer survivors may change drastically over time, through phases of diagnosis, treatment, and beyond.

Finally, in this death-and-illness-phobic, youth-and-beauty-adoring culture, many of us live far from our aged kin and see them rarely, compared to earlier times when we lived with and cared for our elders, so we don't have the daily role models that our ancestors did. We don't have the opportunity to learn how to be care providers.

So what's the point? The point is to inspire you to imagine; to illustrate what may help or hurt; to provide a range of possibilities and contexts so that after considering your audience and taking focused time to think, you can determine what's most beneficial to the person you want more than anything to support. The purpose is not to dictate right and wrong, because what soothes one may scrape or stab another. The purpose is to provide general guidelines and principles of compassionate communication; to help you realize that what comes out of your mouth is born in your history, and you can keep it there if you want. As the grandmother of etiquette, Emily Post, wrote almost a century ago, "Think before you speak—nearly all the faults or mistakes in conversation are caused by not thinking."

Think about these questions before you speak: Do you want to ask someone with lung cancer whether they smoke because you smoked and fear you could get cancer? Are you compelled to tell someone with cancer that you know someone else with cancer who just died, because you're shocked and don't know what else to say, or feel uncomfortable touching her hand and saying something simple like, "It's not fair"? Do you feel a blurt coming fast as a fart because you cannot stay in your own fear?

And before you act, or neglect to act, ask yourself this: do you conveniently become too busy to call or visit because you fear facing a tragedy that could befall you or someone you love?

If you ask yourself those questions, you will surely find the words and actions to show how much you care.

Why don't people with cancer just tell us what helps and hurts?

Why should we have to guess what others want and need from us? Why don't they just assert themselves if we blurt something that upsets them, and ask us to zip it? If they don't want our advice, why don't they just say so?

Many people, whether they have cancer or not, fear hurting the offender, whom they assume meant no harm. Therapist and two-time breast cancer survivor Halina Irving, who has worked with survivors for decades, says cancer patients not only fear hurting others, they lack emotional strength because they are traumatized.

"All this talk today about patients needing to be proactive, well that's well and good, but to ask someone to be proactive at a time they are least able to be aggressive and assertive is very, very difficult because we regress more to a state of dependency."

And in that state of dependency, we often fear that if we confront the offender, they may leave us forever.

Why not just follow the Golden Rule?

On another writing retreat, I found a puzzle of Norman Rockwell's famed painting *The Golden Rule*, which appeared on a 1961 *Saturday Evening Post* cover. It shows some twenty people of different ethnicities, ages, and religions standing together; some with pressed palms in prayer, others holding native tools or sacred objects. Superimposed over the painting, in all capital letters, are the words "Do Unto Others as You Would Have Them Do Unto You."

Once I began assembling the pieces, I could not stop. I yearned to make it fit together, to create order from chaos, to make meaning from bits of seemingly meaningless images. All the while, I admired the beautiful faces—brown and ochre, smooth and leathered—and contemplated the Golden Rule. Like a prayer, I got lost in the puzzle, finally completing it after midnight.

I awakened the next morning, turned over the puzzle box for the first time, and read about the illustration:

"The Buddhists say, 'Hurt not others with that which pains yourself.' In the Jewish Talmud we find, 'What is hurtful to yourself, do not to your fellow man.' And in the Hindu Mahabharata, 'Do naught to others which if done to thee would cause thee pain.'" And so on, through all the faiths.

A few days later, I interviewed Irving. "It's seems so simple. Why don't we just follow the Golden Rule when dealing with people with cancer?" I asked.

"We don't always know what we would want under those circumstances," said Irving. "I think this is the one experience you have to have lived to really know what you would do."

Or, I would add, "what you would *want*."

That's why a chorus of voices as diverse as the faces in Rockwell's illustration will sing a symphony of stories in multiple keys; hopefully, one or more will resonate with you.

What I hope you will get out of this book is not just answers, but also relief and reassurance. Putting yourself in your friend's or loved one's shoes will enable you to step back out, relieved perhaps to face your own familiar problems again. More important, the experience will leave you richer for having truly given of yourself—for having helped someone live. As an added bonus, helping someone else live may help you live as well. A recent study showed that people who showed more compassion exhibited lower blood pressure, heart rate, and levels of the stress hormone cortisol.

Once you have completed the book, you should find it easier to follow Ms. Post's first, last, and only rule:

"Above all, stop and *think* what you are saying!"

And hopefully you will find the strength to say nothing at all, except with your arms, open to embrace a shocked or weakened body, or your eyes, open to acknowledge and hold someone's anguish. Just the fact that you are reading this book tells me that you cannot help but find your way.

Throughout this book you will be a fly on the wall in the lives of people who share a class of disease, but who sport idiosyncratic and sometimes contradictory needs. Although individuals may differ in major ways, fundamentally people are people, and as the Help Me Live Survivor Survey indicates, most of us want the same things: to feel heard, respected, understood, and valued. Most of all, we need to feel loved. "I love you," in fact, are the words survey respondents said they most want to hear.

If you remember just one idea from this book, I hope it will be to think about the person with cancer *and what they may need*, not what you need. It is not about saying what's wise, intelligent, or compassionate. It is about saying what the patient wants to *hear* and what will buoy hope. He or she, not you, is facing the battle of a lifetime—sometimes the battle for life itself.

So when you are faced with the face of cancer, don't look away. Watch. Listen. Think. Comfort. Love. That is what will help your friend or loved one live.

part I:

20 things
people with cancer
want you to know

1:

"It's okay to say or do the 'wrong' thing."

I have brutalized more patients by responding
lovingly and caringly in the wrong way.

—Lawrence LeShan, PhD

WHEN MY FRIEND ALICE WAS about to undergo minor surgery and asked me to take her to the hospital the morning of the procedure, I agreed without hesitation. She was there for me the day I was diagnosed with cancer—her birthday, in fact, which I had forgotten and she did not mention—and throughout my lost-in-space trip through the Cancersphere. She helped create a luscious garden of chocolate mint, rosemary, and thyme in my front yard; brought gifts such as lavender bubble bath to soothe my sorrows; took me for a massage soon after my body healed from surgery but my spirit still ached with dank memories.

Alice explained why she wanted me, of all her girlfriends, to take her to surgery. "I know you can keep quiet—that you won't be yakkin' all the time!"

I awakened at 5 a.m. that June morning, worried and anxious. My cancer surgery almost exactly one year before had frightened me to my core, and Alice's imminent operation took me back to the morning of mine. The thought of losing her was terrifying, and I couldn't seem to shake it, but I knew not to share my trepidation with her. Resigned to a masquerade, I downed two cups of extra strong coffee and set off to face the day with a strong face.

When I reached Alice's home at 7 a.m., I was still buzzing.

"Hey! How you doing?" I asked, eyebrows raised too high.

"I'm okay." Always the polite hostess, Al proffered a cup of coffee.

I should have known better, but I thought gripping a cup might help me get a handle on my fear. Instead, I lost hold.

"I'm so glad I get to be with you this morning," I chirped. "So, how you feeling? Did you see that story on the news last night about the new museum?"

Like a dog wanting to go out to pee, I shadowed Alice from kitchen to dining room to living room, continuing with, "What time do we need to get out of here?" "How long will it take to get to the hospital?" "Should I park in the garage or on the street?"

"Shhhhhhhhhhhhhhhh," Alice breathed out slowly "I need calm. I need *quiet*," she whispered.

I couldn't believe what I had done, knowing what a person going into surgery needs! And Alice had even asked for what she needed.

> *I appreciated honesty and people who said they were afraid of saying the wrong thing. Even when I did, I knew how much they cared.*
>
> —L.C., kidney cancer survivor

Why we blunder

I blundered that morning because, wrapped in my own understandable fear and anxiety, and moving posthaste, fueled by caffeine and a desire to get on with and beyond the surgery, I lacked the consciousness to train my focus on Alice. I was simply not there.

Sometimes we blurt because we feel uncomfortable and gravitate toward tried and true platitudes that are untrue more often than not, but which anchor us in an idealized reality (see chapter 16). Another reason we slip is that in our silence, we feel awkward and think we should gift someone with wise, helpful words. But in fact, as we will see later, and as Rachel Naomi Remen, MD, one of the earliest pioneers in the mind/body holistic health movement and cofounder of the Commonweal Cancer Help Program wrote in *Kitchen Table Wisdom: Stories That Heal*, "Perhaps the most important thing we ever give each other is our attention. . . . A loving silence often has far more power to heal and to connect than the most well-intentioned words."

We may also feel plagued by guilt or shame at the secret relief we feel at having thus far escaped this fate ourselves. Comparative religion scholar Karen Armstrong says it is important we acknowledge and accept that everyone has a dark side, so we can have compassion for others and ourselves. We may also harbor the belief that somehow our friends' suffering is deserved or earned, as Rabbi Harold Kushner explores in his evergreen book, *When Bad Things Happen to Good People.* Instead of accepting these normal and understandable reactions, we may experience punishing anxiety and confusion, causing us again to focus more on ourselves than the person we want more than anything to help.

In any event, no matter why we may err, it's imperative we realize that such errors are not only fully understandable but also wholly forgivable.

Nobody's perfect

Confucius said, "Be not afraid of mistakes and thus make them crimes."

Jimmie Holland, MD, chair of the department of psychiatry at Memorial Sloan-Kettering Cancer Center, is known as the "mother of psychooncology." She said of mistakes, and she has heard about plenty in her almost half-century of practice, "I do think you can say the wrong thing and apologize and it's okay. If you say the wrong thing and realize it and say it with sincerity—'I'm really sorry, I realize that wasn't a good thing to say'—people will forgive you."

One cancer survivor who answered my survey said she realized after later becoming a social worker that her expectations of her loved ones had been too high. "Somehow I thought they should know what to do or say and they didn't always, even though they cared and tried," she wrote. "Maybe what made a difference in my reactions to people was my perception that they were honestly trying to understand how I might feel."

Even when people sustain wounds from gaffes or slights, most realize the speaker's good intentions. A male respondent who answered my survey said that although he had "of course" been hurt by things people had said, he usually noticed and appreciated their efforts more than their words. And he forgave them. Just as important as being forgiven, however, is to practice self-compassion and forgiveness. To neglect to do so may cause you to not only hurt yourself and undermine your own confidence, but to hurt others down the line even more. By feeling fearful, you may hold your tongue unnaturally, adding further distance between you and the person you want to comfort.

"Anytime you suppress what you want to say, you inhibit yourself; you put up a wall between you and the person with cancer you are talking to," said Irving. "And if you have to start watching your words that carefully, you'll run out of words, and its going to become very tense and stilted, and the patient will feel it and will say 'I want people to treat me like me, not just like a cancer patient.'" (See chapter 13.)

Worse, your discomfort may cause you to avoid your friend or loved one, further isolating him when, as we will see in the next chapter, he most needs to know he's part of the herd.

Six words in sequence that never fail

There are six words that, when strung together, can defuse even the most nuclear of emotional energies:

"I don't know what to say."

Why is it so difficult to admit that we don't know what to say, or that we are simply at a loss for words? Often the most vital and honest form of communication happens not through the spoken or written word, but through silence and nonverbal language. Yet we are thinking creatures and problem-solving bridge-builders who want to feel useful and competent. Often it doesn't even occur to us to accept an emptiness of mind, which may know better what a friend or loved one needs.

I can't count how many times I have shared these six words with people who have asked for tips about how to support someone with cancer, and have been met with a resounding "Aha!" reaction. And in talking with other survivors, as well as people traumatized in other ways, they've soundly agreed that often, just hearing "I don't know what to say" removes the lid that allows built-up steam to escape and love to flow unimpeded.

A practice in acceptance and self-forgiveness

A few years ago, when I was approaching a book deadline, I took a writing retreat in the Santa Cruz mountains. On the second morning, I awakened extra early to meet my friend, Den, at his doctor's office, thirty minutes away. A single dad of two, Den had recently been diagnosed with cancer and was about to learn the results of diagnostic tests that would indicate whether the disease had spread. I planned on leaving for the appointment a half hour early to make sure I arrived before he did, but somehow had pushed the alarm clock snooze button and barely had time to wash my face before sprinting out the door.

I knew Den was petrified, and feared letting him down. I also knew that he should have someone with him to take notes, ask questions, and help synthesize information, and that those were skills I possessed. But in the days before the appointment, I worried about my book deadline. Den had told me his pal, Gary, was going along, so I let myself wonder whether my presence was necessary, rationalizing, Maybe I should go the next time, when I can be of more use.

I knew from having a friend with cancer how terrifying it can be. I kept that in mind when people said inappropriate things, and forgave them of course.

—S.D., breast cancer survivor

What?! My friend and the father of two children I love like family was to learn that morning whether his cancer might kill him. And I had a skill set I couldn't be sure his friend Gary possessed.

Thanks in part to my friend Ellice, one of the most ethical people I know, who had earlier exhorted, "*Of course* you should go with Den!" I silenced my inner whiner and drove down the mountain at 7:30 a.m. Although I knew I had a good grasp on words and actions that would best help Den, I suspected that along the way I would likely say something wrong. So I pledged to stay as silent, attentive, and loving as possible.

Den and Gary walked into the reception area minutes after I did. When Den saw me, a look of relief and joy warmed his fear-frozen face. We enjoyed a mighty hug and made small talk, although nothing seems small when you're awaiting test results.

"How you doin,' man?" Gary asked Den.

"A few pins and needles here."

"That's understandable," I said, proud to have caught myself before saying, "Don't worry," which might have sounded dismissive.

> *Doing nothing or holding back is worse to me than doing too much or saying the wrong thing.*
>
> —A.D., chronic myelogenous
>   leukemia survivor

A nurse led us to the exam room. Den sat on the exam table, shoulders hunched and hands between his knees. I felt an impulse to put my arms around him. I obeyed.

The oncologist knocked softly before entering. Ready with writing tools, I scribbled almost every word he said. The good news was there was no sign the cancer had spread; his scans were clear, and his labs showed no evidence of tumor growth. But the doctor referred Den to a surgeon at Stanford who might remove the remaining abdominal lymph nodes to prevent the possible spread of residual cancer cells.

As the doctor rattled off instructions for Den—pick up his CAT scans from the hospital, PET scans from another department, and labs from yet another location—I wrote them down. Smiling reassuringly, the doctor said, "See you in four weeks. And I do believe you're going to be okay." It doesn't sound dismissive coming from an oncologist.

Gary and I stood up, walked over to Den, still seated on the exam table, and put our arms around his shoulders. The three of us shared another bear hug. After a few seconds, Gary said, "We gotta stop; I'm getting excited!" and we howled with laughter. "That's why men can't hug," I said, clicking my tongue.

Gary seemed to know exactly what to say to Den. "What I heard the doctor say is that you're going to be okay." Den replied, "Yeah, but this really sucks." "Yeah," agreed Gary, "and I didn't really get excited!"

More laughter. "You guys up for a cup of coffee?" I asked. My work could not have mattered less at that point.

I tried not to talk about my own cancer, knowing that most newly diagnosed patients prefer to talk about their own experience rather than hear about others,' but found myself subtly giving advice. While passing by a newspaper rack on the way into the café, I glanced at a headline about the beheading of an American soldier in Iraq, and said, "When I had cancer, I stopped reading newspapers and watching the news." "You didn't want any more bad news, huh?" replied Den. And I realized that was about me, not him.

Gary brought up the subject of living healthfully. "Well, I guess it's a good idea to do what we should all be doing anyway—eating right, exercising...."

"Yeah, when I had cancer I started meditating for the first time in my life," I added, and then wondered, Am I advising Den about what he should and shouldn't do? Is that what he needs?

We had already given him what he needed most: our love. And some laughs. Gary told a joke. I asked how work was going. Gary asked about the kids. We talked about funny movies.

I was immeasurably glad that I accompanied Den that morning. Though I may have made some "wrong" moves, and I of course fretted about them on the ride back to the retreat center—Did I talk about myself too much? Did I share too much information about a supplement I take? Why did I say how great I thought it was that he wouldn't have to go through chemo knowing that, when you're diagnosed with cancer, the only great thing is the possibility of being cured?—I had only good intentions.

I hoped for the courage and humility to apologize to him for my errors in speech or judgment, and knew that he would forgive me.

Three good things that have come from not doing the "right" thing

Benjamin Franklin wrote, "The greatest question in life is, 'What good will I do with it?'" We can certainly choose to use our mistakes for good. I know of three women who did this, turning errors of omission or inadequacy into gifts for many others. Therapist and cancer survivor, Susan Halpern, MSW, neglected to visit a sick neighbor. The regret that stayed with her was the partial impetus for her book *The Etiquette of Illness*, an outstanding resource for friends and caregivers. The second woman, Debbie Sardone, owned a house cleaning service, and after turning down a woman with cancer who couldn't afford to hire her, had an immediate change of heart. Though she could not find the caller, she founded Cleaning for a Reason, a nonprofit that helps provide free house cleanings to people undergoing cancer treatment. I am the third woman. My regret that I could not better support my chronically depressed mother has helped drive my sincere wish to help others.

It's almost inevitable that you will say or do something that could be misconstrued or in some way disturb someone with cancer. Just remember that you only use the misstep to do good, but also that it is never too late to admit to your friend or loved one that the most caring words escaped you—that you are sorry for any possible transgression—and that you want more than anything to help.

What has far more potential to devastate is when you are so guarded and frightened of infelicities that you stay away from people who need you more than anything. As author Peter McWilliams wrote, "To avoid situations in which you might make mistakes may be the biggest mistake of all."

What's most crucial is to simply be there.

2.

"I need to know you're here for me, but if you can't be, you can still show you care."

It's the friends you can call at 4 a.m. that matter.

—Marlene Dietrich

THIS CHAPTER IS THE NEXUS of this book because it concerns the kernel, the seed, the center of our very being.

First, I feel it is safe to say that all of us want to believe that our friends and family will be there when we need them most—and that our deepest fear is that they will not be.

The harsh truth, that too many of us who have been diagnosed with cancer have discovered, is that some people *will*, while others will *not* be there for us. As the philosopher John Churton Collins said, "In prosperity our friends know us; in adversity we know our friends."

In the following pages, the diverse tales will show how some people have shown up, and suggest why others may have disappeared. If you happen to be someone who has a difficult time being there in person for someone else, we will illustrate how you can still help, or at least mitigate the pain your conspicuous absence might cause.

〓〓〓

Marching to mastectomy

Sarah was a grandma when she told me her life story and why she always thought she would die young.

"I was born here, but my dad died right after I was born and my mother took me in a laundry basket on a train back to Ohio," she explained to me over lunch at Zza's Trattoria on a sunny autumn day. "Then she died of breast cancer. So I always lived with this kind of fear in the back of my mind.

"The day I outlived my mother—my mother died when she was fifty-one—I bought the best bottle of champagne in the whole world, got rip-roaring drunk by myself, and said 'Yeah! I got beyond it!'"

> *What really helped was a friend who would just come by and sit with me, never telling me what I ought to be doing, just being there.*
>
> —N.N., large cell neuroendocrine lung cancer

But eight years later, Sarah learned she had breast cancer. "I had the galloping kind—the kind that was going fast," she recalled. "And they said they wanted to do a mastectomy, and I said, 'Why don't you just take them both off and I won't have to worry about being lopsided?' My mother's cancer had traveled to the other side within a year, so why not get them both taken off at once?"

Sarah's candor came as no surprise. A half hour earlier when she walked into my office, she had hugged me as if we were childhood pals. Then she clutched the bottom of her tightly knit red-and-white-striped sweater, lifted it up, secured it with her chin, and pulled her prosthesis-filled bra up over her chest.

"See? They're both gone," she exclaimed, smiling so widely that her crow's-feet stretched almost to her hairline.

"Wow," I said, disarmed. I had never before seen a chest bare of breasts and nipples in the flesh, blank like a shield.

Face to face at the restaurant, she detailed her harrowing but hopeful march through Cancerland, while air as warm as her smile blew through the open window where we sat.

"I was absolutely terrified," she began. But my family just pulled together. It just makes me cry to think about it."

Her thirty-five-year-old son, who lived in a nearby suburb, did research for her. Her thirty-three-year-old identical twin daughters were there for her, too, arriving for their mom's surgery even though they had careers and families to care for.

"The [doctors] wanted me there at six in the morning," Sarah said, smiling. My kids came from Los Angeles, and my son had had T-shirts made."

Emblazoned on them was "Marching, marching to mastectomy."

"It was so wonderful; we all wore them, holding hands, walking to the hospital."

Sarah's surgery went well, but soon after, she learned the cancer had spread to her lungs and she would need to have one of her lobes removed. Just when it seemed things could not get worse, they did.

"My husband was diagnosed with prostate cancer the same day I had my lung surgery, and everyone in the family said, 'You gave it to him, Mom. That's what happens when you sleep with somebody—he gets it, too.' And then we started saying, 'Yeah, we want to go to every floor in the cancer center—breast, lungs, prostate—how many more floors are there in here?'"

Sarah was as present for her husband as he had been for her. But some people don't have loving spouses or family members as dedicated and committed as hers. And some say they do not have family at all.

Why people disappear

"I have NO family. Dispersed and dysfunctional," Abby wrote in an email. She began her story saying that her friends helped tremendously during her two bouts of breast cancer. One girlfriend went camping with her after chemo, and, in a tender gesture, offered to rub her bald head. "It was good strokes, both physically and mentally," Abby noted.

"The most touching thing was when I was diagnosed, one of my best friends asked, 'What time are we going to the hospital?' She stayed with me through the operation, without my asking."

But there were two people who didn't stay with her at all. "I was the most hurt by my closest friend, who did the least. Ditto for my brother. He couldn't deal with the disease."

I know that my being sick scares you. It scares me, too. Don't stay away from me because of this. We don't have to talk about it. Just be here for me.

—R.C., melanoma survivor

My husband and daughter were there for me anytime I needed them, never judging my response to things, just loving me.

—D.B., endometrial cancer survivor

Abby said she could understand her best friend's reaction, because the friend had lost her mother to cancer. And she realized she couldn't change her brother. But she does believe her loved ones could have lessened the sting of abandonment.

"What would have eased the pain of these unsupportive people would have been a verbal or written message that they're not equipped to deal with my cancer," wrote Abby, perhaps trying to muster compassion herself. "Not everyone can deal with life-threatening situations, but to ignore a person without an explanation tears at the heart. This is not the time to add stress."

Abby's siblings and best friend added stress with their unexpected absence. "My best friend, who I've had since high school, didn't call me until probably three months into my treatment, and then I had to call her," she said sadly. "Now, I knew she knew, but I think it was just really hard for her to face. Finally I had to break that barrier. I had to see if this was a rejection of me, or if she was just having a tough time facing it. It was more her having a tough time facing it, but in your mind you kind of think, 'Am I like a leper that people don't want to see'?"

If I'm there for you, will I catch your cancer?

When I recently conducted an Internet search, "Is cancer contagious in humans?," 3.9 million hits came up. You'd expect that question from a child, but most of the links I sampled didn't concern children. And as one of the Help Me Live Survey respondents wrote, "Because I had leukemia, people wanted to know if I was contagious."

The American Cancer Society clearly states on its website, "Scientific studies of cancer causes show that there is no way cancer can be considered contagious. If cancer were contagious, we would have cancer epidemics just as we have flu epidemics—cancer would spread like measles, polio, or the common cold. . . . This is not the case."

Cancer is not contagious, but, like leprosy, it can instill primordial, sometimes unconscious fears of isolation, disability, and agonizing death.

Some treat people with cancer as if they're contagious, superstitiously suspecting that that they may catch it themselves. Hence they disappear, or find excuses to stay away, whether or not they realize why they are doing so. I recall someone asking me one time, "Why do you know so many people with cancer?" Was it implied that I was helping to spread the disease? I wanted to say, "Because I don't run away from them," but instead, just shrugged.

Bay Area Tumor Institute Director Barry Siegel says some people rationalize being absent because they convince themselves they don't know what to say and are better off keeping their distance.

I loved to hear, "I'm here whenever you need me."

—S.B., breast cancer survivor

"We think [the patients] are already damaged goods. But all we've done for them at that point by staying away, is we've cut them off from the social interaction that makes us people."

Siegel, whose nonprofit agency provides information, referrals, and support groups, used to teach philosophy. "Aristotle said man is a social animal. Now we're going to cut him off from being a social animal because we're frightened that we're going to hurt his or her feelings, when that's really a time when greater social intercourse is needed."

Why some people really can't be there

"There are some people who can't deal with bad news, they can't deal with sick people, they can't deal with people who are losing their jobs, and their range is rather restrictive," explained psychologist Paul Ekman, who has worked closely with the Dalai Lama, and authored more than ten books on nonverbal communication.

"When you say 'can't,' do you mean 'unable' or 'unwilling' to deal with it?" I asked, having always considered it a matter of choice.

"Unable to. I think most anyone would make that choice if they could, but these people can't deal with it, they just aren't psychologically able to do it."

Dr. Ekman explained that some people have little capacity for emotional empathy, or rather, feeling what another person is feeling. Others lack cognitive empathy, meaning the ability to understand intellectually how someone might be feeling. Still others have little compassionate empathy, the desire to help.

Others, of course, are pregnant with compassion. But unlike a woman with child, a truly compassionate friend may be difficult to identify until you're ill. Some people I barely knew seemed to appear out of the ether to help. That's not surprising when you factor in emotional vulnerability. It was easier for me to support peripheral friends and relatives with cancer than those closer to me, such as my father. It hurt more to see him suffer, and because my fear of losing him was so acute, I became easily mired in the quicksand of terror.

My family (three siblings and my mother) wouldn't call or check in on me. They kept saying, "I don't know what to do." I would say then, "Why not ask me?"

—C.T., breast cancer survivor

But regardless, the reason some people aren't there for their friends and loved ones, according to Dr. Ekman, is that they just don't know what to do. "They don't know what they're supposed to say. Illness used to be a part of everybody's life, as part of their extended family, since they were a child—when they had aunts and uncles and grandparents around—but now, by the time friends get seriously ill, they aren't prepared."

Dr. Ekman said some people fear they will make things worse for the patient if they allow them to talk about how bad things are. "But really it just makes it worse for them, not the sick person. So you have to hope they have a lot of good fortune in their lives," he said and laughed, "because they won't be able to deal with their own misfortunes when they occur."

His face turned serious as he continued. "We like to think that life is controllable and predictable, but the only things for sure are death and taxes . . . and with taxes, you know when they are going to occur."

How to be there without being there

Being there need not necessitate face-to-face or even voice-to-voice contact, and often the patient may reject such contact, but still need and appreciate support. Such was the case with Ancil, a retired executive who volunteered as a patient administrator for a health-care institution. When he was diagnosed with tonsil cancer, he was treated with both radiation and chemo in the hospital where he worked.

"He was very self-conscious about his appearance, as the radiation had left him with severely burned lips that turned black," wrote his daughter Melinda. "The only people allowed to visit him were immediate family and his priest."

But his coworkers wanted to do something for him and felt helpless when he refused to see them. "They called me to ask what they should be doing," continued Melinda, "and when I posed the question to him, he said that what he really wanted was the *New York Times* to read each day. His coworkers took turns buying him the paper, clipped personal notes of encouragement to it daily, and then left it at the nurses' station for delivery."

Ancil was thrilled; it took his mind off what he was dealing with.

"He was back at work within a few months. I often think that having a cheering squad of colleagues so close to him made a difference."

You will find myriad other creative ways to show you care in part II, but for now, keep in mind that just a brief note, voicemail, or text can mean the world to someone with cancer. What matters is that patients know you care, that they matter to you, that your relationship matters, and that you are there to support them in deeds, gentle words, or loving, attentive silence.

Neglect is just as painful as harsh judgment words, especially when it comes from people I have supported in tough times.

—J.B., lymphoma survivor

3.

"I like to hear success stories, not horror stories."

My words fly up, my thoughts remain below.
Words without thought never to heaven go.

—William Shakespeare

IN A 2010 *VANITY FAIR* ARTICLE, "Miss Manners and the Big C," author and political and social commentator Christopher Hitchens shared what happened to him at a book signing shortly after he was diagnosed with esophageal cancer. A "motherly looking woman (a key constituent of my demographic)," he wrote, engaged him in the following conversation:

She: I was so sorry to hear you had been ill.

Me: Thank you for saying so.

She: A cousin of mine had cancer.

Me: Oh, I am sorry to hear that.

She: (*As the line of customers lengthens behind her.*) Yes, in his liver.

Me: That's never good.

She: (*With those farther back in line now showing signs of impatience.*) But it went away, after the doctors had told him it was incurable.

Me: Well, that's what we all want to hear.

She: Yes, but then it came back, much worse than before.

Me: Oh, how dreadful.

She: And then he died. It was agonizing. Agonizing. Seemed to take him forever.

It got worse from there. She ended her pitying saga by sharing that the patient's family disowned him and he died alone.

Nightmares can end as comedies

I have to urinate. Looking for the restroom in a dark, crowded, unfamiliar restaurant, I walk through a fluorescent-lit hallway, heading for the door at the end. But the sign reads, Restroom for Staff Only. Back in the dining room, a waiter points the way to the public ladies room. The sign on that door: Out of Order.

I look at the dots, lines, and numbers glowing in the darkness: 4:15 a.m. As I awaken, I try to recall details of the dream, but only the feeling of desperation remains. I get up quietly, trying not to awaken my husband, David.

As I regain full consciousness, examining my tired eyes in the mirror above the bathroom sink, it all comes back. Not the dream, but the events of the evening. Not the tastes and textures that delighted my mouth during dinner, but the harsh acidity that remains six hours later.

Earlier that night we dined at an Italian restaurant, becoming more relaxed with each course, from Apertivo to Antipasto. The owner came to the table to ask about our meal so far, and we seemed to make his day with our "perfectly seasoned" praise. I asked how long he had been in business.

"Twenty years," he said. And then, as if ripping open a wound, he bared his heart, sharing that he and his wife had opened the restaurant, but she died of cancer four years ago. "I still miss her every day," he said softly.

"I'm so sorry," I said reflexively. Then added, "I had cancer, too."

"What kind?"

When I told him, his face augured the imminent gushing of grief.

"That's the kind of cancer my wife had," he began. "The first time she had it, she had surgery and was fine. The tumor was contained. No chemo, nothing. But eight years later, it came back," he continued.

> *Many people want to make it seem like they can relate to what you're going through, so tell you about people they know who have had cancer, but it does not comfort you.*
>
> —H.L., adult Hodgkin's survivor

Having had lung cancer myself a year and a half earlier, I pleaded in my mind, Enough! Please stop!! But I remained silent, breathing in his pain. I also sensed David's terror. Seven years from now, would he be speaking those words about me?

"It was so horrible," the restaurateur agonized like it happened last month. "The cancer had spread everywhere. She was coughing up blood; she died within a year."

The waiter arrived with a cup of minestrone, and I attempted to breathe in its aroma instead of the owner's acrid pain, but I could not divert my eyes from those of the widower. Trapped in his suffering, the fear flowed through me with the same force as the pain that poured from him.

After I was first diagnosed, we were boating with my mother-in-law and sister-in-law. They spent the entire afternoon telling me about everyone they had known that had cancer, and telling me the details about how many of them had passed away. It was made me feel terrified.

—A.L., breast cancer survivor

Finally he left, and David and I looked at one another, eyes round. After a moment, we erupted in nervous laughter at the insanity of enjoying a candlelit dinner in a glaring spotlight of raw suffering, while considering the possibility that my cancer could return and kill me within a year.

We ordered a second glass of Chianti and by the time we finished the tiramisu, the terror of the widower's horror story was almost forgotten.

But now, six hours later, I stand wide-awake in the bathroom, the horrifying words and images persisting in my mind's eye. I scurry back to the safety of our bed. But I cannot sleep. I listen to the ticking clock, asking myself where—whether—I will be a decade from now. David awakens, as if he has heard my thoughts.

"You okay?" he asks.

I consider protecting him, but I so badly need comfort myself that I begin to cry, quietly, and tell him my worries.

He holds me and whispers, "You're going to live." I tell him how much I love him, and get up to write so he can go back to sleep. I know I will not be able to rest until I exorcise my fear through words.

But I don't journal, instead I huddle in the dark living room, crying softly into knees hugged to my chest. The sky lightens and the doves coo outside. I relax my legs onto the floor and Franny, our heat-seeking-missile cat, pounces into my lap. Our bagel-and-cream-cheese bassett hound, Belle, pounds her tail against my chair, and I stroke her long, soft ears.

Eight years. Is that how long I have? How to fill that time? What can I do to survive longer?

And why did that man have to tell me that story, knowing I had lung cancer and could face the same fate as his wife?

"His need to tell the story was greater at that moment because he's still carrying the grief," explained therapist Halina Irving, when I interviewed her the next day. "His need to talk about it was greater at that moment than his ability to think about you and how that would make you feel." She said the reason it frightened me so much was that my diagnosis was fairly recent, and it can take years to rebuild a sense of safety.

When I first heard this tall, slender woman with a slight German accent on *The Group Room*, a nationally syndicated radio show for people with cancer, I was immediately struck by not only her intelligence but also her deep compassion.

"We have to have a special tolerance and understanding of anyone who has suffered a loss," she said, "because the imperative to tell the story is their survival, is their healing, and that's why I believe in grief work and grief counseling. We live in a culture that doesn't allow for that."

But sitting across from Irving in an office beautifully decorated with antiques and matted and framed heartfelt notes from patients, I still felt confused about what happened with the restaurateur who lost his wife. Why did I awaken in the middle of the night? Was it simply that I needed to urinate, or did terror preclude my peaceful sleep? And what could be done

> *There is absolutely no way that a person who has not had cancer can fully understand the feeling of absolute vulnerability and terrorizing fear that occurs when you hear the diagnosis of cancer. It was the first time in my life that I had really thought about my own mortality.*
>
> —J.M., prostate cancer survivor

to prevent such incidents in the future, besides keeping my health history under wraps?

Irving told me, simply and emphatically, that anyone who is not grieving, as the restaurant owner was, should hold his or her tongue. Instead of imparting advice to me, she shared her thoughts based on her own trauma, including a grim cancer diagnosis and debilitating treatment. For her, it's been almost two decades. For me, it had been just two years.

> I couldn't stand listening to people tell the horror stories of this aunt who died of colon cancer, or that sister-in-law's struggle with lung cancer that she lost, "Poor dear!"
>
> —D.B., colon cancer survivor

"The way you're existing now is the way I believe I existed, which is what we all do because we couldn't live otherwise. We go into some kind of denial—that it [dying of cancer] will not happen to us—and we push away the fact that it might happen to us, because if we thought about it we couldn't go on living. It would be too terrifying." (Indeed, a recent study of more than two hundred people with lung cancer in the Netherlands showed that those with moderate levels of denial, or those whose denial increased over time, not only suffered less anxiety and depression but also had significantly healthier social lives.)

"When someone tells you about another person who has died of lung cancer—when I hear of a woman who has metastatic breast cancer—it shatters our denial, and it pulls us back, *whoosh*, right back to that moment of diagnosis and then treatment, when we felt most vulnerable and most in danger," said Irving. "After [so many] years, it still happens to me, and anyone who tells you that they don't feel that is either lying or their defenses and their denial are so powerful because they're so terrified that they're not able to allow themselves to feel."

Irving assured me that I would survive the frightening stories I will hear, that they will even make me stronger.

Success stories

After actress Dana Reeve, the wife of actor and advocate Christopher Reeve, died of lung cancer on March 8, 2006, I read too many hopeless headlines and heard too many dismal and frightening lung cancer stories and stats, and badly needed hope. So I wrote to my cousin Judy Goldwasser, asking her to retell a story she had shared with me over lunch a couple of years earlier.

Judy responded immediately: "The person who had the lung cancer was another cousin of mine, and it was discovered (somewhat advanced as I recall . . .) when he and fellow med students were examining each other as part of a course. I know he had surgery, not sure what else. His wife, a somewhat cute, spoiled young thing immediately left him because she didn't want to deal with it, but he recovered, became a doctor and has practiced in upstate New York in a small town since he graduated medical school. He happily remarried long, long ago and remains so—and is now somewhere in his mid-seventies, I'd guess. Hang on to that one because you will do equally well."

That story meant more to me than any amount of reassurance I could have received, even from an oncologist, whose words carry considerable heft.

Survivors need and love success stories, with one huge caveat: the circumstances must at least match those of the survivor. For example, a woman with breast cancer will likely only be encouraged by a survival story of someone of similar age and with an equal or more advanced stage of cancer. This means that it would behoove you to find out your friend's exact kind of cancer—there are more than two hundred, and even ones that share the same name, such as leukemia, may differ markedly. But, even knowing that, we sometimes just can't help stuffing our foot in our mouth. One lymphoma survivor who answered my survey said an acquaintance blurted out to her, "My friend just got diagnosed with lymphoma, her prognosis is good, Oh, I'm sorry, I know you have the bad kind."

> *So many people brought out stories about people they had known with cancer. Or they brought out stories of their own aches and pains. I was not in the mood to listen to all of this.*
>
> —I.S., prostate cancer survivor

Something else to be mindful of: it may take several success stories to mitigate the impact of one horror story. I collect hopeful tales and keep them tightly guarded in my heart, just in case. You might consider taking up such a collection yourself by visiting online communities and requesting such stories. You might also read some of the comments posted by frightened, worried patients, because knowing

> *I liked hearing stories about survivors and that it wasn't a death sentence.*
>
> —B.H., lung cancer survivor

how to compassionately treat someone who is traumatized comes more naturally to one who can put himself in another's shoes.

If you do, you will find that the first emotion most people diagnosed with cancer experience is terror—not only of death and difficult treatment but of being abandoned because they feel so angry, confused, and out of control that they say and do things out of character that are sometimes hurtful.

4.

"I am terrified and need to know you'll forgive me if I snap at you or bite your head off."

Some situations are so bad that to remain sane is insane.

—Friedrich Nietzche

TAKE A MOMENT AND THINK ABOUT THIS: remember when you were a child, and how your imagination went wild when you were afraid. Shadows hid monsters. Creaking floorboards conjured visions of evil. Your adrenaline coursed, readying you to fight or fly the coop. As an adult, I had no idea that, just before my family was to fly our urban coop for a country vacation, I would feel a coursing of adrenaline like I'd never felt before.

We had been planning our getaway for almost a year. During the previous spring, David and I had driven the ninety miles from our home to the small Russian River resort town of Guerneville to look at vacation homes to rent with our dear friends from Oregon, Barbara and Peter and their daughter, Isa. For the first time, they were coming to the Bay Area for our annual summer vacation together; the past four years we'd traveled north. We feared their sticker shock—everything in California seems to cost twice as much—and we wanted to make sure we found a place that was economical and beautiful.

I anticipated our annual getaway with alternating giddiness and serenity. How I looked forward to a week without makeup or pretense of any kind; long, wristwatch-free walks through the ancient redwood forests; nothing to decide but which pleasures to enjoy. This summer we would feel the hot sand-and-pebble river beaches beneath our feet. I looked forward to the laughter of children and teens as they inner-tubed in the clear water and rode the Octopus and Ferris wheel at the amusement park nearby.

But amusement was the last thing on my mind when, just four days before our vacation, I heard the words, "It's cancer." The sensation was unlike any I had ever experienced. Terror shot through me like lightening. Panic permeated my body as well as my soul. My heart felt as it if would pound through my chest wall.

> *Mostly, I wanted those close to me to just hug me and understand how frightened I was. I didn't need them to say anything, especially overzealous words about my future that sounded superficial.*
>
> —T.P., leukemia survivor

I couldn't wait to get the cancer-ridden lobe of my lung removed from my body, but while awaiting test results to try to stage the disease, I learned that I would not undergo surgery for almost three weeks. So we decided to take our vacation, and I looked forward to it even more, partly because Barbara ranks among the most compassionate people on the planet, and I needed compassion as surely as the breath that had been punched out of me earlier that week. I knew Barbara would listen to me, and that her sensitivity and wisdom would soothe me as deeply as a massage, which she treated me to later that week.

When I mentioned to another friend, Angela, how excited I was about spending time with our Oregon friends, she asked, "Do you think you'll really be able to relax, knowing you're facing major surgery?"

"I'm sure I will," I assured her. I had recently begun to meditate, and knew I would also find peace in the aromatic pine and eucalyptus forests.

"Okay," she said, dropping her eyes. After a few moments of silence in which the refrigerator buzz grew as loud as a mosquito in my ear, the conversation changed course. But her question stuck in my mind. I felt dizzy. Upset. Angry. Scared. Confused. Why did she have to ask me that? I wondered, growing more furious and frightened as the seed of doubt took root.

The angel on my left shoulder assured me that Angela meant no harm. "It was just a question. It'll be okay." The demon perched on my right shoulder pricked me with its trident. "Angela is right. You *will* have an awful time.

Postpone the trip." The angel countered, "You need this, it's exactly what the doctor ordered." "Are you kidding?" asked my devil. "You'll probably have to come home midweek for more medical tests."

I thought I was going mad. How could one simple little question make me a whirling dervish of good versus evil, faith versus fear?

We took the trip and, though I felt like a burn victim whose skin no longer protected my nerve endings, the love of friends and family shielded me. And although I did have to drive back into town midweek to get a bone scan, having Barbara and David along was anesthesia to the psychic pain I feared I could not endure.

己己己

"When anyone's diagnosed with cancer, we cannot overestimate how vulnerable we become; how hard it is to think clearly; how anxiety distorts our sense, our judgment, our ability to think clearly," said Halina Irving. "Whenever we face a terrible crisis, a terrible loss or a threat to our lives—trauma—we regress emotionally and we need to be taken care of. Think of a child who has a trauma, whose mother goes away to the hospital for instance: a child who has given up the bottle asks for the bottle again; a child who has been toilet trained needs a diaper again. It's a temporary regression, but it has to do with the trauma of a diagnosis, which robs us of that false sense of safety that we had that there was a future."

Said one melanoma survivor who responded to the Help Me Live Survey, "My wife just let me cry, and often cried with me. In my worst moments of uncertainty, I was little more than a small child emotionally."

Most people with cancer become more vulnerable, sensitive, and highly attuned to all stimuli, especially soon after diagnosis, even if they appear to be handling it well. "What cancer patients face is this other dimension of reality in which we have this constant awareness that we may not be able to go on living," observed Irving. "It's like being chased by a tiger in the woods. That's what it feels like."

> *Suddenly, you're a mere mortal and the possibility of death is real. There is also a sense of betrayal: how could my body give out on me this way?*
>
> —J.J., uterine cancer survivor

Wake Forest University Medical Center Professor Richard McQuellon, PhD, and Michael Cowan, PhD, wrote in their book, *The Art of Conversation*

Through Serious Illness, about what they term *mortal time*. They use the phrase more "to capture the experience of being acutely aware of one's own mortality than to describe a particular period," but it applies to "the experience of human beings confronting the prospect of death. This confrontation can stimulate intense feelings, a flurry of thoughts, and erratic or unusual behavior. . . ."

Everyone's moods swing, but many who have had cancer experience frequent and intense emotional bungee jumps. Though we may react one way one day, we might react differently to the same words or actions the next day, week, or month. Just as our moods change, so do our needs. Joanne, who was diagnosed with advanced cancer three years ago, said during chemotherapy it didn't bother her if someone asked about her plans for the next year. But at other times, it would scare her to think twelve months ahead because she didn't know if she would be alive.

Personalities can jump from Jekyll to Hyde in seconds. Mine did, especially before my surgery. I felt so unnerved and emotionally off the charts that I knew my father and my stepmom, Judy, must be warned. They had just arrived for a three-and-a-half-week stay. After only a few minutes of catch-up chat in the kitchen, I told them there was something I wanted to talk about. In retrospect, that must have terrified them. But I wasn't thinking about them.

> *Please know that we are scared, and for someone who lives alone just a simple hug can fill us more than a great dinner out. They say of the five senses deprivation of touch is the most severe. A sincere hug or holding of one's hand can release the fears we've been holding and allow ourselves to feel cared about.*
>
> —D.K., melanoma survivor

"Let's go into the living room," I suggested, and took several deep breaths. My thoughts and feelings muddled together like primary-colored paints turned dirty brown. I was frightened at what I was about to say, at my depth of fear, that my words would make my parents stand and leave the room, the state of California, and me. Forever.

"I am more terrified than I have ever been," I said. "I don't expect you to understand, because I don't think you really can unless you've been through this. But I am so afraid, I can't even describe it.

"So, I want to warn you," I continued, voice quivering. "I may be overly sensitive now. Unpredictable. I may snap at you. I may say things I don't mean. And I just want to tell you that and ask you in advance to forgive me and to please step lightly."

The fear on their faces relaxed into relief as they realized I was not going to tell them I had six months to live. Judy, deeply caring and compassionate, said, "Of course," and stood to give me a hug. Dad did, too, and the three of us shared a moment of love during which I may have forgotten for a few nanoseconds that I had cancer.

I don't know why I was able to speak so candidly that afternoon. Where did I get the courage? Perhaps it sprang from survival instinct or, more likely, a deep well of trust. Whatever inspired me, others may not have the time, opportunity, or inclination to initi-

I loved it when my friends and family tolerated my occasional unexpected sarcasm. It wasn't like me to be that way at all, but I wasn't always myself."

—R.R., melanoma survivor

ate such conversations with their loved ones. And too often, people with cancer snap or blow up without knowing why, or before they can consider that they may be transferring their anger about cancer to whomever happens to be close by at the time. As one twenty-year-old survivor commented in the Help Me Live Survey, "Don't take what I say personally. It's most likely the drugs that are making me say what I am saying. If I'm being a bitch, don't bitch back unless it's really out of hand."

Don't give up on us

When Diana and her fiancé, Baruch, struggled with the demands and dangers of his numerous tumor surgeries and rapidly changing state of health, their moods changed rapidly, as well. How they wanted to interact with their many supporting and loving friends changed frequently, too.

"Sometimes you want them to call two or three times and check in; sometimes you want them not to call back. I'm thinking of my two best friends," said Diana. "When I was mean, they showed up again the next day. When I was needy and weepy, they were there."

Being there, showing up, means trying again and again when loved ones shut you out.

"You know how some people ask you, 'Do you need such-and-such?'" said Melissa, who had been treated for both breast cancer and melanoma.

*I just needed them to understand
that I was not at my best mentally
and emotionally and to be patient
with me.*

—T.U., prostate cancer survivor

"And so you say, 'I'm taken care of that way,' and then they stop asking after that one time? But I had another friend that I'd say no to, and she'd still offer because she knew there would come a time when I would accept it.

"She would ask each and every day, 'Do you have someone to take you? Are you eating dinner tonight? Are you taken care of this week?' and I really liked that." Melissa added that this friend had survived cancer herself. Not surprising. People whose loved ones have helped them live know what it takes to help others on the path of healing.

Loaded words that can make us snap

Certain words and phrases almost automatically induce trepidation, terror, anxiety, and dread in cancer survivors. *Mortality rate*, *metastases*, and *recurrence* have implications that can stop you like a snake on a hiking trail.

Harvard psychology professor Dr. Ellen Langer wrote about a word heavier than an ounce of gold: *remission*. Her mother died of breast cancer at fifty-six, but before that, her oncologist declared that the disease had gone into complete remission. In an essay published in *Psychology Today*, Langer questioned what that meant.

"If two people go for a checkup to see if they have cancer and one never had the disease while the other person is in remission, the test results look the same," she wrote. "Psychologically, however, 'remission' may be very different from a 'cure.' Language has the interesting property of being able to increase and decrease our perception of control. Different word choices can direct our thoughts about a single situation in many different ways.

"Consider the way we deal with cancer. If somebody has cancer and the cancer goes away, we say it is in remission. The implication is that the same cancer will recur."

I remember the first time someone asked me whether my cancer was in remission. My stomach sank as if I had flown into turbulent skies. It was soon after my surgery, and it hadn't occurred to me that I might have to go under the knife again. I had focused so intensely on my tests showing the cancer hadn't spread that I had not allowed myself to imagine that I might again hear, "You have cancer."

Langer wondered whether the word *remission* contributed to her mother's death. "Being in remission means that we are waiting for 'it' to return. . . . Psychologically, this may lead us to feel defeated. For each new cold we beat, we implicitly think, 'I beat it before, I can beat it again.' If the cancer comes back, however, we think, 'It is winning. I am just not as strong as it is. . . .'"

"It is clear that giving up impairs people's physical health and keeps them from wanting to survive. Why exercise or take medication if one is likely to die soon anyway? Did cancer kill my mother or was it the language that we used to describe cancer that led her to give up?"

> *Don't assume you know what end of the spectrum I am on any given day. You don't have to know a thing about me or about cancer because all you have to do is ask.*
>
> —S.D., breast cancer survivor

Most of the time, it isn't life itself that lies in the balance, yet certain words clearly shape our perceptions and can cause knee-jerk reactions. One acquaintance asked me how I was progressing after my surgery. To me, diseases progress, while health improves. Someone else asked if I was maintaining. To me, *maintaining* implies an imminent drop, as in airspeed. When I read in an obituary that journalist Faith Fancher "succumbed" to cancer, it angered me, because *succumb* implies that she consciously allowed the cancer to win. Perhaps she did surrender to death and hopefully passed peacefully, but I knew her to have a fighting spirit, and I don't think she would have liked anyone implying that she made the disease her master. (For more specific examples of potentially dangerous words, see chapter 30.)

Though subtle, these semantic differences enlarge under the magnifying glass of illness. But that doesn't mean they'll ignite a piece of paper even under such a focused light. And if a flame does erupt, it can be extinguished with tenderness and understanding. As medical doctor and cancer support group leader Jeff Kane said, "Not taking someone's anger personally is a *skill* deserving of development." Please work on developing that skill. Please forgive us. And let us know it's okay for us to express our fears. Listening to us—truly hearing us—can help us live well almost more than anything else.

5.
"I need you to listen to me and let me cry."

Remember that silence is sometimes the best answer.

—The Dalai Lama

"KEEP YOUR EYES AND EARS OPEN AND YOUR MOUTH SHUT!!!"
He moved his mouth with the speed and precision of a karate kick, shocking, disarming, and terrifying his young charges. Although none were yet twenty years old, the boys—some gangly, some shaped like the McNuggets they chomped—looked like men in their uniform-blue prison garb. But their faces belied sheepishness, fear, and shame, as if they were about to get their first haircut. In fact, most had just gotten their first buzz cut, and robbed of their hair, may have been able to relate to someone undergoing chemo. But unlike people with cancer who lose their locks through no fault of their own, these boys were losing their mullet cuts as partial payment for their transgressions.

It was the 1980s, and I was making a documentary about prison overcrowding. We visited a Georgia boot camp to see how corrections officers were discouraging teen criminals from violating the law as adults, when their crimes would exact a higher cost.

The crew-cut corporal told me later in his maple sugar drawl, "It sure gets their attention." Sure did, especially since they had to drop and do one hundred push-ups if they didn't comply. But because most of us don't live with such a threat, how do we learn to keep our eyes and ears open and our mouth shut, in other words, to truly listen?

Telling it like it is

For an answer, I turned to Jeff Kane, MD. I had just read his masterpiece of compassion, *How to Heal: A Guide for Caregivers*, which clearly and lovingly communicates the nuts and bolts of caregiving, which often comes down to this: just listening.

I drove almost four hours across the hay-colored Sacramento Valley and through the Sierra mountains to spend just twice as many hours with this man and a group of people he accompanies through their private hells.

I felt like I had truly entered hell when I opened my car door and walked through the parking lot of the Summit Medical Center. The heat of the pavement baked through my shoes, and although it was October, the air was sauna hot.

Dr. Kane was about to lead a cancer support group, and I was to meet with him beforehand. I made my way to the featureless meeting room, crowded by a large square Formica table, and within a few minutes a tall man with tightly curled hair speckled like gray river rocks walked in. He offered me a kind smile that revealed an endearing vulnerability. We talked for barely ten minutes before members of the support group began to dribble in early, eager to start. The fluorescent lights in the room rendered all complexions pink and blue, but you could feel the warmth of friendship as the room grew loud with conversation.

I never felt that people were "hurtful," but I did get the impression that a lot of time they didn't want to hear about how sick I was feeling from chemo, or how tired I was. I didn't expect them to do anything about my nausea or fatigue, I just wanted them to listen and understand.

—A.D., breast cancer survivor

"Okay, let's check in," Dr. Kane interrupted, his voice raised just enough to get their attention. After introducing me, he turned his gaze, head slightly tilted, to each of the eight men and women around the table.

"How have the last couple of weeks been?"

Harold, a flame-haired man to my right, two heads taller than me sitting down, bellowed in a baritone, "Doing okay." A long pause.

Dr. Kane lowered his chin to catch Harold's downcast eyes. "How's your family situation?"

The group knew that Harold's sister recently died of cancer, and Dr. Kane suspected it brought up fears and anger buried in the eight years since Harold's own diagnosis.

"I ignore everything on both sides," Harold said with a laugh, referring to certain members of his family that he does not get along with. More silence. "I gave up on them a long time ago." More silence.

No one's eyes left Harold as he explained a recent visit to his dermatologist about a rash on his shoulder. "My thoughts immediately went to cancer." Heads around the table bobbed affirmatively, understanding that when you've had cancer, each bump, lump, or headache can seem a harbinger of cells run amuck. Harold's dermatologist examined the rash then asked about the scar on Harold's midsection. Harold told him he had lung cancer and had a lobectomy years ago.

> *Cancer patients are aware of the fact that cancer does have a tendency to come back. When the patient verbalizes this fear, don't minimize it or trivialize it. Be supportive.*
>
> —J.K., lung cancer survivor

"Well, this rash is harmless," the doctor declared. "You're not paranoid [that it's cancer], are you?"

Harold shook his head. "I told him, 'You get lung cancer and see what it does to your paranoia level!'" Everyone laughed together at their own seemingly unfounded but wholly understandable fears. The group loved sharing, with impunity, whatever they wanted, not having to worry about worrying their spouses.

"That's what I love about coming here," Harold said, looking fondly from face to face. "I can tell you when my fingers have been bothering me and no one gets upset. My wife does, though."

Dr. Kane checked in with each member, many who had a long history with the group. Mitchell, a gastroenterologist, said he might not see everyone for a while since he would soon fly to Boston monthly for an experimental cancer treatment with a new drug. "My eight by ten centimeter mass will be removed first," he explained clinically, adding softly, "I met a woman on the Internet who has the same thing; the drug didn't work for her after one year."

No one said a word. They didn't tell him everything would be okay. They just listened.

Opening an oyster

Over coffee later, Dr. Kane explained that his support groups work because they not only facilitate listening, but also acknowledge and accept suffering.

"Part of the skill is just recognizing that [as the listener] you are experiencing pain. You're absorbing pain from this other person, but it's not going to damage you. It's not like you have your hand in a fire. It won't damage you as long as you recognize it, inhale, drink it in, and then exhale it out—let it go." I thought of the restaurateur's horror story and how I neglected to take that last step, to exhale out his pain.

Everyone needs to acknowledge and release pain, Dr. Kane said. "You just get it out, drain the abscess, and finally, you're at acceptance. And that's when the work starts."

It amazed me that Dr. Kane worked with such a wide range of individuals in his group, from a cabinetmaker to a fellow MD to a sixty-eight-year-old near-hermit who was given a year and a half to live eight years ago. "[Most of] these people are standard middle-class folks," Dr. Kane said. "They don't know from meditation or therapy or anything. I don't have a contract with them. Their doctors say, 'Go to the support group.' That's means a lot of people whining to each other, as far as they know."

Dr. Kane explained that he probes them gently, at first. Not everyone feels comfortable in the group, so he talks about how unusual this kind of conversation is. He encourages them to talk about that and then, if they are ready, to talk about themselves. He asks them, "How is it for you?" Sometimes they answer with vague, tentative responses, and he asks them to say more. As they relax, they sometimes share things they haven't told anyone before.

"You know Anne Lamott, who writes about writing in *Bird by Bird*? It's what she calls 'the really shitty first draft,'" said Dr. Kane. "They just blurt something out. It's something they don't want to say or may have never said. They're uncomfortable saying it. They're not really familiar with what they're saying. And you listen well enough to allow them to say it.

"Like their first draft might be anger at you. They don't really mean that. But it's anger and you're handy. And so can you stay around and say to them, 'What's that like?' 'You're a rotten son of a bitch, really,' they might say. 'Tell me more about that,' I ask. And they just go on."

Dr. Kane makes a point to ask each group member what's most disturbing about having cancer. That initially angers some, but when they follow the conversation to its logical end, which can take a while, most conclude, "It means I'm going to die."

"Okay, so what's new about that? I could have told you you're going to die," Dr. Kane says. "What bothers you about dying?"

"Well, I have business to finish," some might say.

"Really? What sort of business?" After thinking more about it, one group member said, "I want to reconcile with my kids."

"What's really bothering her about her cancer is the cancer's telling her she might die with unfinished business," Dr. Kane explained. "And now she knows what it is. And she knows what to do about it. There's nothing I need to do. I can't tell her. My role is just to ask the questions that lead her into the center of it."

Hold my hand

"Where did you come from?" I asked Dr. Kane. Although I knew he practiced as an emergency room physician in Berkeley for ten years before learning how to heal versus "cure" people, I wanted to understand how he got from there to here. He sees his journey as an act of grace.

"I just went into the ER one day and I was dissatisfied with it. It felt like I'd been trained to be an engineer—that I was just operating a turnstile—people come in and I fix them and kick them out again. I wasn't sure what my values were; all I knew was that it didn't feel right."

Dr. Kane quit his job, taught philosophy at a community college, and became a yoga instructor. But he returned to conventional medicine as a healer, founding the support program at Sacramento's Sutter Cancer Center and Grass Valley's Sierra Nevada Cancer Center, and later becoming the director of psychosocial education. The winner of the "Heroes in Healthcare" Lifetime Achievement Award, he has led support groups for more than three decades, frequently speaks to physicians and other caregiver groups around the nation, and trains peer navigators and others who support people with cancer. Having seen him in the support group situation, he still seemed most like a therapist to me.

"You can think of it as therapy," he said, "but I really think of it as friendship. How would a friend behave with you? A real friend would draw out your feelings."

Still the scholarly philosopher, Dr. Kane further elaborated on why he sees himself as a friend rather than a counselor.

"The model I use is Virgil and Dante," he said, referring to the *Inferno*, the story of Dante's journey into hell from the *Divine Comedy*. "The illustrations always show Virgil holding Dante's hand—always, in every picture, leading him to hell. Dante's always horrified, confused, enraged, and frightened. And each time, Virgil is just there holding his hand, encouraging him, supporting him.

"It's different than the healing of the doctor-patient relationship, which is more vertical. It's just being human—and not having to fix it."

> *Allow your friend to say how they are really feeling and don't feel that you have to "fix it." Listening is enough.*
>
> —S.B., cervical cancer survivor

Asking questions and listening to answers seemed to come easily to Dr. Kane. But he admitted that he still struggles to be a friend. As a trained physician, he sometimes wants to ask what a patient needs, even when he knows that will not be helpful. He suspects it is because he wants to stop them from talking, because they're telling him about their pain at a time when he has had enough.

He said that what usually helps someone most has little to do with words or actions. "What everyone tells me is that as soon as they get diagnosed, all this stuff begins to accumulate next to their bed: books, diets, crystals. The stuff just comes. This notion that you can help by giving something is noble. It sounds altruistic, but it doesn't work. What really helps is to bring something out of the person: 'Tell me how you're suffering.'"

Crying out

I'll never forget the first time I saw my father cry. I was maybe five, eating breakfast at our glossy-red 1950s style glass-topped kitchen table. Dad was always cheerful in the morning, but I recall his wide smile falling flat when his steaming cup of instant Folgers spilled into his lap as he reached for the *St. Louis Globe Democrat*.

"Oh, my God!" Mom screamed, bolting to the freezer for ice.

Dad didn't scream, but his eyes scrunched up and filled with tears, face wrinkling in agony. I cried, too.

"It's okay, Sweetie," Mom cooed. "Daddy will be okay," she said, tattooing my forehead pink with her lipstick. She led me by the hand into the bedroom she had appliqued with teddy bears and bunnies. But even those happy creatures were no comfort; I was panicked and confused, and sat motionless on my bed. A few minutes later I heard my parents laughing in the kitchen—they were probably trying to figure out how to explain to me what happened. No explanation was necessary. I knew all I needed to know: "Daddy was okay!"

My next sight of a grownup in tears was more shocking and perhaps more terrifying. The school principal came into our classroom and beckoned our teacher, Mrs. Coffey, into the hall. When she returned, head bowed and silent, oblivious to the chatter of fifth-graders, we quieted ourselves. We saw something that challenged our idea of reality: a teacher transformed by tears into a vulnerable human being.

Sometimes someone would ask how I was and when we started talking cancer, they changed the subject. That made me feel horrible.

—M.L., breast cancer survivor

"Boys and girls," she said, "President Kennedy has been shot."

She wept, as did adults everywhere that day, unashamedly. Perhaps for the first time, children witnessed a flood of tears on television, and may have wondered, "How can we be safe with so many grownups crying? Who will protect us?"

There was one leader I knew would protect us: Jackie Kennedy. She didn't cry.

"First Lady Holds Strong for Nation," read the headlines. I remember puzzling over how she could control her tears. It seemed impossible that anyone could keep up such a strong front if she were really suffering. Surely she must have ached deeply enough to weep. But she never did, at least not publicly, as far as I knew. She was a model of strength; she symbolized our nation's fortitude in the face of fear or foe.

Forty years later, almost to the day, another headline shattered my sense of reality: "Diary Reveals Grief of Jackie Kennedy."

An Associated Press article reported: "To a grieving nation, Jacqueline Kennedy was stoic after her husband's assassination. But over games of tennis with a priest who counseled her, she apparently revealed her feelings, including thoughts of suicide."

The priest left behind his typewritten diary when he died, which included recollections of his private conversations with the First Lady.

"I'm so bleeding inside," she had told Rev. Richard McSorley.

The Associated Press article continued: "The release has raised questions about the propriety of a priest keeping notes on private discussions." But, to me, it raised questions about keeping a stiff upper lip and sucking it up. I was relieved that Jacqueline Kennedy had not only experienced, but also expressed her grief.

Six months after the assassination, she wrote Rev. McSorley saying she would never get over her loss. But what if she had revealed her grief publicly? What if she had talked candidly about her feelings of hopelessness? Would that have made it easier for her to recover from her loss? And would it have made it easier for a woman named Ruth to talk about her feelings forty years later?

Telling your story makes it real

Like the former First Lady did when she was alive, Ruth loves tennis. She also enjoys exercising her intellect as much as her body, and after working as a physical therapist for decades, Ruth recently earned a master's degree in philosophy.

"People think philosophy is so esoteric, but to me, philosophy is everything," she said. I tend to agree, having earned a BA in philosophy. To this day I still "love the questions themselves, like locked rooms . . . ," as poet and philosopher Rainer Maria Rilke exhorts in *Letters to a Young Poet*.

Ruth continued, "Philosophy comes down to the very core of what you think about yourself as a human being and how you relate to fellow human beings; to me, that is the most integral thing there can possibly be in your life." But there may be one thing even more integral: life itself. Ruth came to that realization when she was diagnosed with breast cancer.

She underwent a lumpectomy and had just begun radiation treatment when we spoke.

"I'll just go on with life as usual. If I have to deal with something, I will."

But she was more philosophical when she spoke about the experience of diagnosis itself.

"It's a very surreal experience being diagnosed with cancer. You feel totally normal, and all of a sudden somebody's saying you have this very potentially life-threatening thing. After a week or so, it was almost like I was shell-shocked, and my tendency was just to go home and let it kind of filter in." But she realized what she needed to do was talk about it.

"I was reading this one article for a philosophy class, and what this person was writing was that the boundary between the real and the unreal is much more blurred than what we would, in a normal sense, or intellectually, want to countenance. It talked about how important the narrative is—that is, the storytelling. That's what makes something real."

Ruth explained that she needed to tell the story of her diagnosis in order to believe it herself. "It was really important for me to talk about it over and over again. It was like the talking about it somehow allowed me psychologically to let it become a part of my reality. And I started thinking about it and realized that I've experienced that throughout my life. I remember when I got engaged. It didn't seem real until I told people about it. Or when I was pregnant . . . you don't really feel it in your body, so it's not real until you talk about it and draw other people into that reality with you. Then it becomes part of your life history."

Although Ruth acknowledged that it was sometimes painful for her to talk about her diagnosis, it was also therapeutic. And once she allowed herself to talk about cancer, it somehow became less frightening. The problem was, some of her friends didn't welcome conversation about her cancer.

"They wanted to express support, but they were also afraid that they were going to make me sad. And so it would be sort of like, 'Let's not talk about it because I don't want to make you sad.' And 'Let's just do something happier.' And I certainly wanted to go out and still laugh and have fun with my friends," Ruth said, "but I think people should know it's okay to talk about it and it's okay if I cry, because those things all help me get through the process. When you're holding it all inside and working it over in your mind again and again, it becomes ten times worse."

Research supports the importance of crying. A study by William H. Frey at the St. Paul–Ramsey Medical Center showed that emotional tears contain two kinds of stress hormones, which, as they leave your body through your eyes, create a calming effect.

I wondered what it was like for the former First Lady to keep her tears to herself. As a nation, releasing our tears collectively helped us cope with the assassination of her husband. We talked about the loss for years, and still do. His death became part of the national narrative, and talking about it helped us heal. Did Mrs. Kennedy's lack of a public disclosure preclude her healing?

President John F. Kennedy's inaugural speech was justly famous for this line: "Ask not what your country can do for you, but what you can do for your country." In honor of him and his bride, consider this: now is the time, when your friend or loved one has cancer, to ask what you can do for her or him. You may hear the answer, "Just let me talk."

How to listen

The Women's Cancer Resource Center (WCRC) is a nonprofit that provides information and support at no charge to women throughout the San Francisco Bay Area who are impacted by cancer. It sponsors numerous support groups, including a posttreatment group I attended, and fields hundreds of calls weekly requesting information and referrals. But often, the callers just need to talk. It's imperative that whoever answers, knows how to listen.

Students from the University of California at Berkeley sometimes intern at WCRC to earn credit toward their degrees. WCRC Program Director Dolores Moorehead trains them to answer the phones.

"A lot of them are very concerned about saying the wrong thing. And my feeling is that you can't say the wrong thing," Moorehead explained to me. She said people sometimes say less-than-ideal things because they become uncomfortable with silence. "But if you're a really good listener, you listen, and the silence is okay." Moorehead advises her interns, "You listen to the person; you allow them to have their silence. And you think before you respond. And it doesn't mean you know the answers."

Christina Puchalski, MD, of the George Washington Institute for Spirituality and Health, an organization working toward a more compassionate health-care system by restoring the heart and humanity of medicine, calls that "listening without an agenda." She trains her students, who are studying to become physicians, that being present emotionally with patients is as integral to healing as treating them medically.

"When a patient comes in and we're discussing what they've just been told by their oncologist, it's in my mind to have a script, which is 'Now I've got to make sure I order the blood test, I've got to make sure I get them to this next [medical] level.' I have to have that in my mind, sure, but then I'm not really listening if I'm [operating from] my script.

"Really deep listening is letting go of my script for awhile. Sure, I'll get back to it. Sure, I'll make the appropriate connections and help them navigate, but I need to stop that for a little bit to just be where they are. Sometimes deep listening is silent."

Like Dr. Kane, Moorehead believes that problems often arise because people want to solve problems, and therefore provide fix-it answers. But often, women who call WCRC simply yearn for listening ears and an open heart. They need someone on the end of the line who can keep their eyes and ears open and their mouth shut.

True listening means focusing completely on the speaker—keeping your eyes trained on her, turning off your cell phone (a real compliment to anyone you're with!) and otherwise limiting distraction, and resisting the urge to interrupt. (Note: For more listening tips, see chapter 31.)

Though many people with cancer need to tell their stories and openly shed tears, some say they sometimes need to listen to *others* and may even welcome hearing about others' woes since it takes their mind off their own. But it's both considerate and polite to ask permission before heaping your troubles onto someone burdened by cancer. It's a good idea, in fact, to ask permission before saying or doing a host of things to someone with cancer. Although, as Stewart's Law of Retroaction posits, "It is easier to get forgiveness than permission," failing to ask permission can cause a lot more suffering.

6.

"Asking my permission can spare me pain."

And this is one of the major questions of our lives: how we keep boundaries, what permission we have to cross boundaries, and how we do so.

—A. B. Yehoshua

SUSAN CHERNAK DRINKS A LOT. That's how she describes herself, often to people she has just met. Not only does she disarm with that statement, she ups the ante when she explains why. Most don't know whether to laugh or cry. Susan had cancer of the mouth, and most of her salivary glands were removed, so to keep her mouth hydrated she must sip liquids.

She and I sipped coffee together just after breakfast in a softly lit dining room of a hotel. A best-selling author and sought-after speaker, Susan was a presenter at the Cancer as a Turning Point conference across the street, which I attended in search of inspiration and stories. She delivered both.

"I was working with a wonderful firm when I discovered a lump under my tongue," Susan began, looking down and moving her fork in a little arc on the table. "After surgery and a round of chemotherapy, doctors told me I was just fine. But eight months later, it came back.

"The well of fear was so enormous," she recalled, stopping the fork abruptly. "And I had been a person so easily swayed by the influence of others that I became intuitively aware very early on in the process that I needed to watch what was told to me." Susan has always known how sensitive she is. "Other people's words have governed me my whole life. Am I okay? Do my parents need me to be like that? Then all of a sudden you've got cancer. Well, you know, are they telling me to be dead? I'll be a good girl and be dead!"

Susan tried to control others' words, including the dentist who broke the news that her tumor was malignant. "I said, 'Don't tell me what kind it is. I'm not ready to hear it.' My dog had died of malignant melanoma, and I didn't want to hear the word 'melanoma,' because she had a tumor in her mouth just like I did. And my dentist respected that."

> *I didn't like having meals delivered, unless I was asked on that day because some days I hated looking at or smelling food.*
>
> —M.D., breast cancer survivor

But not everyone respected or understood her sensitivity. After her tumor was removed, one young hospital resident told her she had a ninety-two percent chance of recurrence within a year. "And he was saying, 'You're doing really well now, but we've really got to track you.' Well, why? 'Because you have blah-blah-blah.'"

Susan interrupted him and asked where he got the ninety-two percent figure. "He said it was in all the statistical data. And I said, 'Yeah, but didn't you also just tell me that I'm probably the only woman my age with this in the entire county? So I don't fall into that statistical data, do I? So my case could be way better or way worse!' And he said, 'You know, I hadn't even thought of that.'"

Susan warned him, "You watch that. Watch it, because I hear you. And new patients hear you."

I felt like applauding, but instead lauded her as a great teacher.

"No, I'm just a bully," she laughed. "He was good, and he caught on." But not everyone did. In fact, the person who probably loves Susan more than anyone else didn't seem to realize how much power her words wielded.

"Mom wanted me to come to her house and do my recuperation there. I had a sense that I needed to be alone. . . . I did not need my mom's fear on top of me through that. But Mom wanted to take care of me."

Though Susan told her mother she wanted to stay at her boyfriend's house since he worked all day and she could enjoy some much-needed rest and solitude, her mother insisted. "I called your dentist up the other day," Susan's mom began, ominously. "He told me about cancers like yours. He told me that what will happen is that it will just keep coming back and it will eat away your tongue and it will eat away your jaw . . . and then you'll be dead. And will your boyfriend take care of you then?"

Susan sighed, making the arc again with her fork. But she smiled crookedly and peeked up, eyes twinkling. "I said, 'Good-bye, Mom,' and I hung up the phone. She has no memory of ever having said that. I think that catastrophic illness can bring the crazies out in people. And they'll blurt out their worst fears onto you."

Susan's cancer created a well of fear for almost everyone around her. "I was almost expecting to take care of everyone else. I remember my mother once saying to me, sobbing on my shoulder, 'You have to tell me you'll be okay.' And I said, 'Mom, you're my mother. You're supposed to be telling *me* I'm going to be okay. So if you need to hear I'm going to be okay, you need to find it from someone other than me. Go talk to your friends and ask them to tell you.'"

"Asking" is a key concept for Susan. Few of us ask permission before dumping our feelings onto someone else. But doing so is particularly important when dealing with someone who has cancer—someone who may be at their very weakest and can't support the weight of their own terror, much less someone else's.

Susan drew on her experience with animals, which she wrote about in her best seller, *Animals as Teachers and Healers.*

"Nature works by the law of consent and permission. Animals and trees don't spend their time running away from situations that aren't good. They spend their time using all of their senses to gravitate to what attracts them. If something does not attract them, they leave. If a seed tries to grow in a place where the sun is not consenting, it will die. The more consent you have in your life, the more you will thrive."

Susan said animals go to a place and watch to get a sense of its safety, if the water's clean, or if there's good food. If animals don't stop to obtain consent, so to speak, it can cost them their lives, because they can miss that a cougar is waiting to pounce.

"Part of consent is asking permission," Susan said. "People don't ask permission for anything. I know that because I'm a real bullish person. But when I go into nature, if I ask permission to be there, if I ask if I'm welcome in this place, I start to feel a kind of yes or no. I realize how important that process is for thriving and living in balance."

Susan wishes that, when she had cancer, her friends and family had asked for her consent before acting. "You know, like, 'Do you want to hear treatment options? I've been looking into this.' And I could have said yes or no. Or if they would have asked, 'Can I talk to you about my own fears?' I could have said 'Not today.' Or, 'Yes, I would love to hear about them.'"

Her own painful experiences now inform how Susan behaves with others. When she meets people who they have had cancer, she assumes they are newly diagnosed. "I never take the next step unless they invite me to take the next steps," Susan said. "I just have this vision that tomorrow, if everyone in the world started asking for permission . . . the world would change."

Asking permission to share the news about someone's cancer

In the summer of 1995, Ronald was creating masks for the *Sesame Street* television show in Minneapolis and had just won a grant from the National Endowment for the Arts to hold mask-making workshops in homeless shelters in the San Francisco Bay Area, where he grew up and where his parents still lived. He had also started working as a commercial actor again. At thirty-one years old, he was living his dream. But in one moment, at a lunchtime audition, he woke up and witnessed a reality worse than any nightmare.

"I was in a big casting room and I started to feel funny and a woman was walking toward me, and you know how when a record is played backward? That's what it sounded like, and the next thing I knew the paramedics were looking down at me and asking, 'Are you alright?' and they rushed me to the hospital, put me in an MRI and said, 'You have a brain tumor.'"

Ronald flew home to San Francisco.

"It was such a shock. I remember talking to people on the phone and hearing only an empty silence on the other end. People were floored that someone they cared about had this, and they didn't know how to respond to it."

His mother helped and coped by researching the disease. His father took a different tack. "I remember my father would talk about it a lot with people, and I did not like that at all. And it was really hard to get through to him." A private person, Ronald told his father he wanted to keep his condition confidential, fearing people would look at him differently and think, "Oh, there's a dead person." He also worried about possible professional and legal ramifications. "If you're going for a job interview people are going to look at you differently. I mean look at the HIPAA rules. (The Health Insurance Portability and Accountability Act of 1996, or HIPAA, includes privacy rules that prohibit requiring the disclosure of medical conditions.) I mean medical privacy is huge."

Ronald said his father continued to tell neighbors and friends at work, even though he asked him not to. "My dad didn't think he was doing anything wrong. It was a huge thing that was going on in his life."

> *I did not want to discuss my illness with anyone. It was not that I was in denial, but rather to me this was just an inconvenience and this, too, shall pass.*
>
> —W.W., prostate cancer survivor

Permission to visit

It was a Friday afternoon when Dana welcomed me into her spacious Victorian home and offered me a seat at her mirror-shiny mahogany dining room table. And it was a Friday afternoon when Dana got the news that she had breast cancer. (It's uncanny how many people get biopsy results at the start of the weekend, when they have two days to stew and, like a chicken, fall apart before asking all the questions in their minds!)

"I got the phone call from the gynecologist. She told me, 'You have DCIS and it's invasive.' I asked what that meant, and she said 'That means it's not so bad—I'll explain it to you at our appointment next week.'"

Dana was anxious to know more about the disease before then, so she called a causal friend, a nurse, Tina. "Calling Tina was a big mistake," Dana said, eyes wide.

Tina demanded, "You have *what*?

"What did the doctor say, *exactly*?

"Where will you get your second opinion?"

Although Tina asked Dana those questions years ago, they stick in her mind like dried egg yolk. The questions, which were doubtlessly intended to help create a plan of action, did anything but help Dana deliberate.

"I didn't know a thing about breast cancer or tumors. Dana blinked back tears. "I was so shocked when I heard the news that Friday, I don't think I heard half of what the doctor said. And I certainly didn't need the pressure of my friend asking me so many questions; it just made me feel more inadequate."

What Dana did need was a quiet evening at home with her seventeen-year-old son, Chris, and her husband, Steven. "When you're told something like that, you just want to find a little safe pocket and stay there for a while," she said. Although Dana and Steven decided not to tell Chris the news until they knew more, they wanted the comfort of his presence, so they chose a movie they knew he would like. But before she had time to push "play," someone pushed her doorbell button. It was Tina, standing there with her husband, Gerald, a doctor. "I just didn't want you to be alone tonight," said Tina.

Shaken and weakened for the third time that day, but still genteel, Dana invited Tina and Gerald to into the darkened living room. She turned on two table lamps, and went to the kitchen to brew a pot of tea and compose herself. Chris had disappeared, happy for the excuse to phone a friend.

Over tea, the two couples talked not about cancer, but instead chattered about news, recipes, mutual friends—the mundane realities that seemed more surreal than real to Dana that night. Tina and Gerald left about an hour later.

"They didn't make me feel any better. There was no purpose to the visit," Dana said. But it did cleave her family. Although Chris was still home, he was rapt in conversation with a pal. Exhausted, Dana fell into bed, full of dread.

Dana said she not only lost her innocence that weekend, she also lost a friend. "Tina called me and apologized," Dana said softly. "I just said, 'Don't worry about it.' I should have been more honest with her about how it affected us, but I wasn't. I'm just too nice."

To this day, she cannot face her friend. When she sees Tina at the supermarket, she disappears down the next aisle. She even got caller ID just so she could see when Tina called. That night was so painful, she has only told two people about the incident, even though it happened years ago.

> *It was great to have meals made, but only if they asked first. I had one well-meaning friend who decided I should go vegan, and what she made was awful. It was great if they put their names somehow on the casserole dishes because it made it easier to return.*
>
> —A.M., testicular cancer

If Tina had simply called and asked whether Dana and Steven wanted company that night, what was essentially an emotional disaster could have been averted. Dana rues the loss of her friend and blames herself, in part, for not being honest with Tina when she showed up at the door. But many people would agree that the onus lies on the friend to ask permission, especially on a day when patients feel like they've been dropped in the middle of a minefield. In the Help Me Live Survey, in fact, more than half of the people who responded to the question "If there was anything you did not want people to do, please explain," indicated they did not want people to come by uninvited.

Permission to share news items

Soon after I was diagnosed, a few friends sent me articles about new treatments that might help down the road. I appreciated the small doses of hope, and after fully recovering, subscribed to Google news alerts about lung cancer treatments myself. Mostly, the alerts buoyed my spirits, but sometimes, after reading articles that noted lung cancer's mortality rate, I would be thrown off kilter for days or weeks. I finally unsubscribed, but a few weeks later, someone I used to work with sent me an article written by a journalist who was dying of lung cancer. It was decidedly not what I needed to read, and had I seen the headline on a news alert, I would have pushed "delete." But because it was from a friend, I clicked on the link and read the story until tears blurred my vision.

Before sharing news items of any kind with a survivor, make sure you read the article. And then, ask whether your friend would like to receive such news.

Permission to share contact information

A friend told me a story about her young cousin, Alex, who was recently diagnosed with advanced lung cancer. Alex, who never smoked a cigarette in his twenty-five years, had a genetic test to see if he would respond to Iressa, a then-experimental drug. He got good news—he would indeed likely respond to the treatment—and he immediately called his mother to share his excitement. She, in turned, called a friend of hers whose niece, Fanny, had been treated with the drug as well. When Fanny heard about Alex, she asked her mother for his email address.

Fanny then emailed Alex. She wrote that she had experienced awful, and it turns out, fairly unusual side effects from the drug. Instead of instilling hope, the note instilled fear. It also made Alex furious with Fanny's mother for sharing his contact information without asking permission.

Because no one asked for his consent, Alex lost sleep, he said, for several nights. All he wanted at that point was to forget about his cancer—to forget and laugh. That in fact is what most people with cancer say they often need most of all—to get a temporary pass from Cancerland.

I liked it when people would call and make an appointment to come over and see me and call an hour before to check that I was up for it.

—S.T., prostate cancer survivor

7.
"I need to laugh—or just forget about cancer for a while!"

If we couldn't laugh, we would all go insane.

—Jimmy Buffet

AS A JOURNALIST, I SOMETIMES HEARD colleagues toss crude, even seemingly cruel jokes about crimes we were covering across the large cubicled newsroom. It wasn't that my coworkers were wholly insensitive; many of them *had* to form callouses in order to function.

Humor is a common coping mechanism people use when they must regularly witness horrifying situations. Hence the gallows humor we often hear about among police, emergency room staff, social workers, and others who see suffering or tragedy on a daily basis and need to maintain emotional distance and defuse the fear, anger, sadness, grief, or disgust they feel. Although it can be more difficult to see or create the humor in a tragic situation when it is you who are the victim, the ability to lose oneself in levity and laughter is crucial to most of us who have had to cope with cancer. "I need to laugh—or just forget about cancer for a while" was rated the number one statement by the majority of survivors who participated in the Help Me Live Cancer Support Survey.

Jokes were great! I wanted to laugh. And laugh some more.

—D.R., breast cancer survivor

When I had cancer, the disease permeated my entire being, persisting stubbornly in my consciousness: it was my first thought upon my awakening and my last upon retiring at night. Almost more than anything, I needed a break to fortify myself on the long and menacing flight through the Cancer-sphere. I did that through meditation, but also humor. Luckily I had a great role model.

My father, Norman Crasilneck, used humor daily and I'd even venture to say hourly throughout his whole life. He wrote in his obituary (he insisted on writing it himself), "He loved to laugh." He also lied about his death date to make himself a centurion, even though he would only live to eighty-three. But as much as he loved laughing, he thrived on giving others a chuckle and making them feel good about themselves. When he was hospitalized in June 2010 for almost three weeks, I wrote down all the *Normanisms*, as I called them, which he delighted the staff with.

One of my friends is always there with a dumb joke about whatever is going on. I know I can call her up with a problem and be doubled up in laughter within minutes. She got me through the worst parts of treatment.

—B.H., thyroid cancer survivor

When an occupational therapist interviewed him about stairs and other possible hindrances to being ambulatory at his residence, asking, "How were things at home?" he answered in a flash, with a straight face, "She was not beating up on me if that's what you're implying!" Then he quickly offered a perfectly timed smile.

To a nurse readjusting his urinary catheter, which caused him tremendous pain, he said, "You're awful pretty when you're concentrating; I hate you but you're pretty."

He brought out the humorous spirit in others, as well. When a tech spilled Metamucil on Dad, he teased, "I like that color on you better."

"I ordered it specially," she responded with a smile.

And when he left the hospital to go home under the auspices of hospice, he said to his doctor, "I'll be okay. How about you?"

"I'll try," said his petite olive-skinned oncologist sweetly.

"Thank you," he said, deeply serious. "Every time I come to the hospital, I'll ask for you."

Other patients use humor to put their friends at ease. Comic Robert Schimmel, author of *Cancer on $5 a Day* *(*chemo not included): How Humor Got Me Through the Toughest Journey of My Life*, told me when I interviewed him, "Your friends and relatives don't know what to say when they're going to see you in the hospital. They turn the doorknob to come in, and they think, 'Oh, God, what's this going to be like when I open the door?' because they're expecting the worst. And if you make light of it, you let them off the hook emotionally and then . . . they can go back to being themselves around you instead of walking on eggshells or being compelled to be a twenty-four-hour cheerleader."

Although not everyone can make others laugh, most everyone can find or create humor. Cancer survivor Saranne Rothberg says that humor may not just help people cope, but perhaps do much more. Comedy can actually cure, maintains this redhead.

Comedy Cures

Saranne is no stranger to the gallows humor of newsrooms. She was one of the youngest local television anchorwomen in the nation when CBS targeted her for the fast track to network news. She later left news for the world of entertainment, cofounding an independent film company, then started a consulting business. Her eclectic career continued its charmed course as she founded an education nonprofit, then earned another academic degree. Along the way she added "mom" to her resume. Then "divorcée." Then "cancer survivor."

In 1999, at the age of thirty-four, when her daughter, Lauriel, was five, she was diagnosed with stage 4 breast cancer. She wrote in *Coping* magazine that she fractured her funny bone. "I heard 'malignant tumor, surgery, radiation, chemo' and felt as if I'd forgotten how to breathe."

It was a Friday (when else?!—the Murphy's Law of cancer diagnosis), and the doctor said it was too late to assemble his hospital cancer squad. So she found herself with sixty hours to marinate in the bitter brew of the unknown. People typically feel more hopeful when they can marshal energy to battle a disease. But Saranne had the whole weekend ahead of her, with neither a

> *One friend became my Ministress of Humor. She sent me funny postcards, called me with off-the-wall jokes, and even brought another friend in to entertain me during an eight-hour chemo session.*
>
> —B.D., breast cancer survivor

partner nor family nearby to support her, plus a young daughter in tow, to boot. What was she to do?

She came up with not only something to do but, more important, a way to escape. "I had read an excerpt from Norman Cousins's book [*Anatomy of an Illness*]—he was the pioneer of therapeutic humor—when I was in college, and all the sudden this man's life story flashed before my eyes, and at that moment I said to myself, 'If Norm Cousins can do therapeutic humor then I can do therapeutic humor'!"

She headed straight to the video store and rented every standup comedy in stock. (This was before streaming, which certainly would have lightened her load!)

"After I put my daughter to bed, for the next twelve hours I laughed and cried through my whole first night, and in that comedy marathon I found my breath in the laughter, I found hope in the laughter."

She said that when she laughed, she felt less fearful and anxious, and she realized in that distraction that she could use a comic perspective to cope and feel normal.

"When I watched the comedy, life seemed like I never got a cancer diagnosis," she said. "It just seemed fun again."

Inspired by Cousins's work and life and her own experience of the night before, she started the next day with a mission: "I asked my daughter if she'd become my humor buddy," Saranne recalled. "I asked if she would make an appointment to laugh with me every day no matter what treatments I had to go through, no matter what hospital I was in . . . I wanted to have two times a day where we would put the cancer aside and just laugh."

> *Laughter was my salve so any funny books, movies, or jokes were so welcome. Anything that reinforced the idea of cancer patients being victims was counterproductive.*
>
> —N.D., prostate cancer survivor

Saranne made that commitment not just for herself, but also for Lauriel. "I feel a lot of times that children are caught in the cancer crossfire, and as a single parent I was very sensitive to the fact that she have the joy, the wonder, the laughter in her day, and that the weight that the sickness and the fear and the pain of a cancer diagnosis not distort her childhood."

Saranne and Lauriel created a daily "comedy and joy workout," like an exercise regimen. Every night, they sat down with a joke book and read jokes to one another. Then they would each find one that they did not read aloud.

"Then we would go to sleep without telling each other, which is kind of funny because we share everything and now we were withholding. Then in the morning, whoever woke up first would run into the bedroom of the other person and before they could say anything, tell them their joke. So your first moments of consciousness are of humor."

What she and Lauriel discovered was that to appreciate life, they had to seek the joy and comic perspective in any moment. "So we developed these highly attuned antennae, like radar, for fun," explained Saranne. "So the little things in life, like the bullies, like the inability of the chemo nurse to find a good vein—all of those things that happen as a result of growing up in childhood or growing through your cancer journey, they all give you opportunities for comedy or tragedy."

They realized that they could choose joy. "Now it doesn't mean you have to, it just means you have the ability to choose." Saranne said that there were and still are plenty of days when she and Lauriel decide to be in a bad mood or cry or feel sorry for their circumstances. "But it's not because we're being thrown into it; it's because we decide that's the emotion that will serve us for that time."

The pair learned that even when caught in a maelstrom of emotions, they could choose to stop and seek the humor or the lesson. "That is so empowering," said Saranne, "particularly when you're a child or when you feel like your life is spinning out of control."

The day that Saranne received her first chemotherapy treatment she came up with the idea to teach others what she and Lauriel had learned.

"My first thought was to redefine what it meant to be a patient. You have to take chemo sitting down, but I realized the chair had wheels. I thought, 'Get up, girl, shake your thing!' And so I started to travel, patient to patient . . . and ask them if I could give them 'a gift.' Some people were very bitter and they couldn't imagine what kind of gift anyone could give you in a chemo facility. Some people were startled and some people were so thankful to have a break from the monotony that they were very inviting."

What Saranne offered was the gift of laughter. Soon she would unwrap it so thousands of others could share and enjoy it. From her chemo chair, with a cell phone and laptop computer, she founded the Comedy Cures Foundation which, within a few months grew into a full-service organization, offering programs such as laugh-a-grams, and live shows featuring New York City's hottest comics.

"We guarantee that in our show you will laugh at least one hundred times. What we do is we have people observe the state of their body, mind, and spirit before, during and after our show, so that you can see in a very real live tangible way the impact these strategies have on you. It's so powerful, it's mind-boggling."

Saranne said the show works, whether you suffer acute or chronic disabilities, depression, or debilitating side effects from treatments. "No matter if you are a two-year-old or a hundred-and-two-year-old, it works every time."

Because not every patient has the energy to pick up a phone or can go to one of her shows, Comedy Cures teaches caregivers how to help their loved ones find humor. Many friends and family of people with cancer complain in exasperation, "We just don't know what to do." Saranne suggests they say to their loved one, "I'd really like to be your humor buddy." She advises caregivers to share how she, with stage 4 cancer, decided to make an appointment to laugh with her daughter every day, and to emphasize how much it helped.

"Do you know that laughter's really good for you?" she sometimes asks callers and then quotes her easy-to-understand synthesis of the studies on the benefits of humor. (According to a 2006 paper published in *Evidence Based Complementary Alternative Medicine* by Mary Payne Bennett and Cecile Lengacher at the Indiana State University College of Nursing, "While there are results to support a connection between sense of humor and self-reported physical health, it is difficult to determine how this may relate to any specific disease process. And while relationships between sense of humor and self-reported measures of physical well-being appear to be supported by the currently limited literature, more research is needed to determine whether this demonstrates the effect of sense of humor on physical well-being or the effect of physical well-being on sense of humor.")

Saranne said scientists have shown that laughing, and even to some degree smiling and thinking humorous thoughts, can positively impact the mind, body, and spirit. "There's a study that shows that your white blood cell count increases; there's an NG4 killer white blood cell that is known to be very effective in fighting cancer and they've shown that you produce more of those cells when you're laughing."

Saranne also said research shows that laughing one hundred times is equivalent to working out for ten minutes on a stationary rowing machine or twenty on a stationary bike.

She pointed to several studies that show laughter decreases stress hormones. "There's a study that shows that [it is also true] for cancer treatment, and when the immune system is under constant stress, it does break down and you become vulnerable to cancer and secondary infections. So it's important to keep your negative stress hormones low and your positive stress hormones high."

To experience the benefits of laughter, Saranne said you have to laugh out loud. That's one of the skills she teaches. "[Laughing out loud] stimulates your auditory response because you're hearing your own laughter," Saranne explained. Also, laughter is contagious, "so you're creating health and energy and wellness for other people instead of just hogging it for yourself."

I just needed someone to help take my mind off all the stuff going on. I didn't want to think about cancer. So just do things like watch a movie or go for a walk and just talk to them and treat them like you would if they didn't have cancer.

—A.S., uterine and ovarian cancer survivor

As if I'm not convinced enough, Saranne threw in one more study that clinched the sale. "If you laugh on the average every day, you will look on the average eight years younger. You never need a face-lift! You're using so many muscles!"

"If my cancer comes back, I might not live long enough to need a face-lift," I laughed, then apologized for my gallows humor.

"Tumor-humor, gallows humor," she squealed, "I love it! But I'm very discreet in how I use it because some people aren't ready."

Friends and loved ones are well advised to use tumor humor prudently, or not at all.

Glenn Rockowitz, a thirty-something cancer survivor and comedian who authored an outstanding memoir, *Rodeo in Joliet*, wrote in a *Seattle Weekly* article, "How Not to Cheer Up a Cancer Patient," that you should follow the "Jew Rule."

"If you're Jewish, you can make Jew jokes. If you're black, you can make black jokes. . . . Well, the same goes for cancer. Once you've joined the ranks of the dying, you can use all the tumor humor you want. Walking by my office to say, "Hey, Uno! How's your last nut hangin'?" really isn't that funny. Especially since I've never had testicular cancer. Again, do your homework."

> *You can lose your hair, your appetite, and forty pounds that will promptly return after chemo. Just don't lose your sense of humor—it's one of your most precious possessions. (My mom taught me that and a valuable lesson it was!)*
>
> —D.K., sarcoma survivor

Saranne's dream is to transform patients' relationships to their cancer from one of a prison to a place from which you can gain freedom from your pain and fear. That doesn't mean people with cancer shouldn't experience difficult emotions. "The first thing that we suggest in our program, and again it's from our own experience, is that you can't fix it, you can't rescue them. You can allow space for people to really mourn the loss of the body part or mourn the loss of their hair or mourn the loss of quality of life, because you can't find the laughter and the joy if you don't let the pain and the anxiety come out."

Saranne believes the process must be balanced; it must allow time every day for complaining.

"I want my daughter to come home from school and complain she has so much homework, but then stop and get down to business. And so as a caregiver or a supporter of somebody living with cancer, the best thing you can do is give them the space to really mourn what they are going through, but then equally give them the space to have fun."

⊐⊐⊐

Facilitating a temporary furlough from Cancerland for a friend or loved one can be as easy as bringing over a pile of movies or a *New Yorker* book of cartoons or pointing your friend to a YouTube video of a baby laughing; as interesting as signing up for a laughter yoga class with your friend or taking her to a play or movie (but beware of Debbie Downer entertainment); as silly as bringing over a puppy or kitten to play (when appropriate: as always, ask permission first); or as challenging as telling a perfectly timed joke. All of these actions, plus others listed in part II, have the potential to launch a spirit beyond Cancerland. But there is one thing guaranteed to sink a soul in less than a second: popping the balloon of hope that keeps the spirit aloft.

8.

"I need to feel hope, but telling me to think positively can make me feel worse."

Take hope from the heart of man, and you make him a beast of prey.

—Marie Louise de la Ramée

I WAS BORN "LORI HOPE CRASILNECK," but in my early twenties replaced "Crasilneck" with "Van Kirk" after a man as romantic as his moniker proposed. Both John and I were working toward philosophy degrees—he as a graduate student, I as an undergrad. Naïve, idealistic, and madly in love, we knew we would grow old together, watching one another ripen and wrinkle like grapes turning to raisins.

We divorced after just four years. A child of divorce myself, the failure stung like a styptic pencil, and I lost all hope for a lasting love. One thing I didn't lose, however, was John's last name; perhaps it was a way of holding onto the dream. But soon I realized another dream: a career that combined my passion for writing and drive to improve the world. I became a researcher for a television-news consumer reporter, then a reporter, medical reporter, and ultimately a documentary producer and writer.

Because I had built a name for myself, Lori (Hope) Van Kirk, I didn't consider changing it, even though keeping it felt somewhat uncomfortable. But when I was thirty-five, I decided to return that which wasn't mine. I bought a bungalow that had green shutters with pine tree cut-outs, rescued a German shepherd mix with rabbit-soft fur, and dropped "Van Kirk," taking Hope as my last name.

A funny thing happened on the way home from the county recorder's office. Rather than thinking of "Hope" as a chewing gum center in a jawbreaker shell, *hope* now became a defining feature for me. And I needed that. Trapped in an enviable full-time job as a network station staff producer whose documentaries aired during prime time on weeknights, I was burning out after making more than fifteen films about social problems. Although the productions included solutions, they also involved inescapable immersion in other realities—such as homeless families and sleepy-eyed, crack-addicted single mothers. How could I survive even one more project?

Changing my name helped. Strangers, upon meeting me, often brightened up: "Hope—great name!" I would smile as my thoughts turned toward hope.

But once I was diagnosed with cancer myself, I feared there was no longer any hope for Hope.

Holding onto hope

In 1992, I produced a documentary about euthanasia, *Help Me Die. . . .* I could have added the subhead, *A Life-Affirming Look at Death*, because, although at first blush, the subject may seem depressing, most of the terminally ill people profiled—many of whom had cancer—remained hopeful. They hoped for a peaceful death; reconciliation; pain relief; grace; acceptance; heaven; healing. Many of them achieved one or more.

I hoped I wouldn't get cancer. I almost expected to fall victim to breast cancer, because two of my cousins had battled it, so hearing "You have lung cancer" was a bolt from the blue. Even though I smoked in my twenties, it didn't occur to me that I could get cancer almost two decades after kicking the habit.

Once diagnosed, I hoped my friends and loved ones would be there for me; that I would survive surgery; that the cancer hadn't spread; that it wouldn't kill me. Initially, that seemed a tall order. I had a form of chemotherapy-resistant lung cancer, bronchoalveolar carcinoma, which tends to occur in younger patients, nonsmokers, and women. (This was before the advent of newer, more effective treatments.)

I wanted to hear success stories. I wanted to hear stories of people who had cancers similar to mine who were now cancer free, had been so for twenty or thirty years, and were living perfectly normal lives.

—B.B., breast cancer survivor

To cultivate hope, I scoured for strings—success stories—to weave a wick for a candle to illuminate my way. When I did harness the will to light that candle instead of cursing the darkness, some people threatened to extinguish the flame with winds of ignorance and insensitivity.

"Lung cancer! OHHHH, that's *really bad*! My aunt died of lung cancer!"

One would expect those with limited knowledge of lung cancer to make hope-dashing remarks, but I assumed that those who shared my disease would be more sensitive. Yet after surgery, when I attended a small discussion group for lung cancer survivors in the shadow of a tall tree, someone extinguished my hope in one swift breath. I had just shared my story with the group, ending with, "My doctor declared me 'cancer-free' after my surgery."

"Yeah, that's what my doctor said, and six months later they found another tumor," said a bald man tethered to an oxygen tank.

His words played over and over in my mind like the song "Time to Say Good-bye" that I heard the magnificent Andrea Boccelli sing soon after my diagnosis. Why did the bald man say that? Perhaps he saw me as boastful and meant to put me in my place. Maybe he was warning me to be vigilant. More likely, he simply said what popped into his mind. But regardless of why, this truth didn't set me free, but thrust me back into my prison of fear.

Fortunately, I met Joanne two weeks later.

Hope is tangerine and moss green

Only about a year posttreatment, I was still raw from the trauma of cancer when I first spoke with Joanne. I knew that she was diagnosed with late stage lung cancer three years ago, so during the drive to her Sonoma County home along a grapevine-lined highway, I steeled myself for a look into the future, expecting to see a woman ashen and skeletal.

Bushes on either side of the flagstone path leading up to her door bloomed pink. A hanging fuscia drew my eyes upward, and I stopped to take a deep breath before ringing the doorbell. But the door flew open, revealing a woman neither heavy nor thin, with a rosy complexion, auburn hair, and eyes the color of moss on a redwood tree radiating warmth and good health.

"Want to sit outside?" she asked.

A half dozen tangerine-orange geraniums grew near the glass-topped table she beckoned me to on her back porch. An iridescent spiral ornament with a dangling glass bead twirled, and a wooden wind chime clucked. Everything burst with vitality, but nothing more than Joanne. How could someone with stage 4 lung cancer be so exuberant?

It wasn't always so. Soon after Joanne's diagnosis, her doctor told her she had six months to live. "I asked him if I would be around long enough to plan a vacation. 'He said, 'You can if you want. . . .' but the way he said it was like he was programmed for six months, like 'You can do what you want, but who the heck knows?' But that was the important part to me: 'Who the heck knows'?"

Joanne and her husband had squirreled away some savings to landscape their back yard, which grew wild with native plants and tall grasses, but after Joanne's diagnosis, they decided to take a family vacation instead, renting a house in Hawaii and flying their children and grandchildren over for three weeks. She had the time of her life, but upon returning, faced a tremendous challenge as she underwent another rigorous course of chemotherapy. She said it was literally killing her, but her doctor told her she would have to stay on it the rest of her life. Her hopelessness turned to hope when she was put on the then-new medication Iressa®.

Almost three years later, Joanne remained in remission.

"We're going to Hawaii again for Thanksgiving," she said. "My goal used to be to turn fifty-nine and to live to see a cure for cancer. My goal now is to be sixty. Renewing goals is so important. You prioritize. Even though my doctor says I'm going to die from cancer, doctors don't know everything. When you're born you have a number, and that's up when God says so."

⧉⧉⧉

Six months later, I called Joanne. Though fearful that she would be near death or gone, I wanted to know how she was doing, so pushed the buttons on the phone slowly and prepared myself to hear a man's voice.

Instead, I heard Joanne sing, "Hell-owe-owe!"

Still on Iressa, she underwent quarterly CT scans to check for new tumors. So far so good. She told me she would soon board a jet for Southern

California to attend a Lion's Club conference at the City of Hope Comprehensive Cancer Center. I told her how inspiring her sense of hope was to me.

"What else do you have to latch onto?" she asked. "I went back to my oncologist; he's always amazed I'm there. He just has to give me the statistics and the negatives . . . that Iressa can only improve life for three years.

"But he gave me a wonderful compliment last time. He said I was important in his life because I taught him how to hope, and that has influenced his patients greatly. I tell him I can go from one thing to the next; I can hold out and wait until there is a cure."

Joanne considers herself realistic; she acknowledges the limitations she faces, but remains sanguine. "I have a predisposition to look on the brighter side, but when I was faced with the realistic impact of mortality there were two ways I could go. I could either say, 'You're right and I only have this amount of time' and give up control—or latch onto something to give [me] a glimmer, the spark of hope.

"I'm doing absolutely everything I can to survive. When control is taken away, that's the killer."

Psychologist Anthony Scioli, coauthor of *Hope in the Age of Anxiety*, would agree. He maintains that hope is rooted in empowerment and personal control, citing a study with rats that showed that those injected with a tumor solution who had no option to escape an electric shock were 40 percent more likely to develop a tumor than those who could find a way out. Was it the lack of hope that killed the trapped rats? Are rats capable of hope? And what exactly is hope?

Does hope have feathers?

Like love, hope has myriad definitions, yet seems to defy definition. You know when you have it, but you can be hard pressed to describe it. Maybe this is why it has been the subject of so many philosophers, poets, and writers through the ages.

Cicero called hope "the dream of a waking man." Nineteen centuries later poet, playwright, and first president of the Czech Republic Vaclav Havel wrote, "Hope is not the conviction that something will turn out well, but the certainty that something makes sense regardless of how it turns out." Emily Dickinson poeticized, "Hope is the thing with feathers that never stops at all." And Friedrich Nietzche, in describing the myth of Pandora's box, which released all the evils, except hope, into the world, called hope "the most evil of evils because it prolongs man's torment." And then of course there's *Webster's Dictionary*: "Hope is a feeling that what is wanted can be had or events will turn out for the best."

When I speak before groups of cancer survivors, caregivers, and health-care providers about how to keep hope alive through cancer and beyond (see chapter 33), I take them through a brief exercise, requesting they close their eyes, take a few relaxing breaths, and remember a time they were hopeful. Then I ask, "What can you tell me about that?"

Virtually everyone shares not what he or she was thinking, but how he or she felt. Certainly, hope is a feeling.

"Just think positive." . . . hooey! LOL . . . that's it? That's all it takes to cure my cancer? And hey, you try thinking positive after a round of chemo. Not that I was all that negative, but it is so easy to tell someone to "think positive" and walk away.

—T.P., lung cancer survivor

Hope heals

Hope is "the elevating feeling we experience when we see—in the mind's eye—a path to a better future," wrote author and journalist Jerome Groopman, MD, in *The Anatomy of Hope*, a book based on his thirty years as an oncologist. Dr. Groopman believes that hope acknowledges the obstacles and pitfalls along that path, and has no room for delusion, but "gives us the courage to confront our circumstances and the capacity to surmount them.

"For all my patients, hope, true hope, has proved as important as any medication I might prescribe or any procedure I might perform."

In his book, Dr. Groopman shares stories of patients who he believes have thrived because of hope, and a few who have failed to thrive in its absence. He documents studies that show that "belief and expectation—the key elements of hope—can block pain by releasing the brain's endorphins and encephalin, mimicking the effects of morphine. In some cases, hope can also have important effects on fundamental physiological processes like respiration, circulation, and motor function." He cites a study showing that people with asthma, when they puffed a placebo in an asthma inhaler canister, felt their airways open as much as those who'd been given a real inhaler. And indeed, the airways of those given the placebo actually did open.

The lack of hope may impair health as much as its abundance may bolster it. In "An Essay on Hope" from *Inner Fire: Your Will to Live* by Ernest Rosenbaum, MD, and Isadora Rosenbaum, MA, the authors cite a phenomenon called "self-willed death or bone pointing" practiced in Australia among Aborigines, as well as in other South Pacific cultures.

"In such cases, a tribal witch doctor casts a spell similar to that observed in Voodoo . . . causing the victim to suffer paralyzing fear, withdraw from society, and die within a short time. Of course the witch doctor can only be effective if the potential victim believes in the power of the curse." In the same way, said the Rosenbaums, a person with an illness can be adversely affected when doctors and nurses project a sense of hopelessness, or when family and friends cannot hide their fears.

Just because I cried a lot did not mean that I gave up hope and still did what I needed to do to take care of myself.

—R.B., brain tumor survivor

This effect has also been called "The Nocebo Effect"—or "Placebo's Evil Twin," in a *Washington Post* article by journalist Brian Reid. Harvard professor Herbert Benson, MD, president of the Mind/Body Medical Institute, is quoted as saying, "Surgeons are wary of people who are convinced that they will die. There are examples of studies done on people undergoing surgery who almost want to die to recontact a loved one. Close to 100 percent of people under those circumstances die."

Surely, hope and belief are real and formidable forces.

"False hope"

When I was a medical reporter, I produced a story about researchers at Providence Hospital in Portland working on a possible cure for cancer involving monoclonal antibodies. This was more than twenty years before the monoclonal antibody formulation, Iressa®—the medication keeping Joanne alive—was approved by the FDA. Part of the reason I eagerly moved on from medical reporting was that I worried about giving patients false hope by prematurely trumpeting treatments that might never become available.

But what is false hope, really? I asked psychologist Lawrence LeShan, known to many as the father of mind-body medicine.

"There's no such thing as false hope," Dr. LeShan answered. "Hope bears its own validity. False hope is a meaningless hope and a disruptive one. What is false hope?" continued the author of *Cancer as a Turning Point*, who said he has seen dozens of so-called terminally ill cancer patients die not of cancer, but of other maladies, often many years later. "It means the person is not going to get better, which means the other person has a crystal ball and knows more about the subject than God. So anybody [who] says you have false hope is an arrogant son of a bitch. You can quote me on that."

How can hope be false, when it is as much a part of the human experience as birth or death? Therapist Halina Irving, who survived breast cancer twice, believes that people always find something to hope for, such as peace of mind, a better world, or a death without pain.

"People hope naturally," says Irving. "You don't have to tell them to hope. When you work with dying people, it's painful in a way to see how hard it is to kill hope, because they've been given the terminal prognosis— they've been told they're going to die, hospice is on the scene, there is no more treatment. And they'll say, 'I know, I know,' they'll acknowledge it, but ten minutes later they'll say, 'Did the doctor call? Did the doctor look at the last X-rays?' That's hope."

Hope may lift the spirits of people who have received a cancer diagnosis. But it is the freedom to experience all our feelings without being judged, without having to hide our doubts, that makes hope possible.

"If we don't have to spend all our energy hiding and suppressing and repressing the fear and the despair, then there's room for the hope," said Irving. "If they can find someone who accepts [their despair], who understands it as normal and is willing to hear it without blaming them, once they feel that and are allowed to go to the bottom, very naturally they'll start feeling better and start feeling more positive and there will be room for hope."

Isn't the bright side always the right side?

"Good morning, Merry Sunshine! God's in his heaven, all's right with the world!"

That's how my father awakened me when I was a child, and he repeated the greeting with new enthusiasm throughout my life when he called before noon. Fun-loving and almost always cheerful, Dad had a remarkable way of letting go of the past and refusing to fret about the future. Yet when his sister died suddenly at the age of fifty-nine, he became agonizingly aware of the fragility of life, and called his children to invite our families on an expense-paid trip to Las Vegas where, together, we would share a penthouse suite and celebrate our love.

Twenty-five years later, when Dad learned that leukemia would steal his future, he did not let it rob him of his good humor. "I know I'm going to die and I don't want to waste time thinking about it," he said to me, adding, "I'll probably go South the skinniest I've ever been."

Continuing to find the bright side, he said, in all seriousness, "I've had eighty-three wonderful years. Most people don't even get that many."

He helped his health-care providers find the bright side as well.

"Remember me?" asked a nurse who came in to give him his meds.

"How could I ever forget you?!" he responded, flashing a smile.

"He has quite a positive attitude," she laughed, glancing at me.

Dad maintained his positivity and attitude of gratitude up to the very end. When he came home to die, his exceptionally loving hospice nurse, Efe Isaac, asked if he was all right. He quipped, "Compared to what?" When she was leaving, he lifted her hand and kissed it, looking up into her black eyes as he said, "Thanks, now I'm a better person."

When his caregiver, John, turned him in his hospital bed, causing acute pain, Dad managed a joke: "I'll see you in the spring if we get through the mattress," then sweetly added, "Thanks for everything."

No one could have been more positive than Dad. And certainly, his optimism softened the devastating punch of his illness and death for himself and for us. But no amount of positive or optimistic thinking could keep him alive. Howard S. Friedman, PhD and Leslie R. Martin, PhD, reported in their 2011 book, *The Longevity Project: Surprising Discoveries for Health and Long Life from the Landmark Eight-Decade Study*, the "biggest bombshell" of their entire project was that "Cheerful and optimistic children were less likely to live to an old age than their more staid and sober counterparts." Later they explain that "Healthy people are happy but happy people are not necessarily healthy," suggesting that happiness is a result of good health, not the other way around.

If hope is so essential, what's the harm in exhorting someone to have a "better" attitude, or, in other words, to think positively? And what's the difference between optimism, hope, and positive thinking?

Soon after reading *The Anatomy of Hope*, and before interviewing Dr. Groopman, I learned of a new Australian study showing that optimism does not extend the lives of people with lung cancer. This seemed to dispute if not the value, then the power of hope. I asked Dr. Groopman about that, and he replied that the Australian study was flawed for several reasons. With only 179 patients, it was too small to be considered statistically valid. Moreover, it studied optimism rather than hope.

People were wonderful about talking about the future in a natural way. It was helpful because I could see that they were assuming I would be around in the future.

—D.S., lung cancer survivor

"Optimism is very different from hope. An optimist says everything's going to turn out just fine. Hope is very different, it sees all the problems and all the issues you're facing and then it chooses what appears to be the best path based on information."

Anthony Scioli said positive thinking, like optimism, is a mental construct, while hope is a feeling, which makes them distinctly different. The difference can be seen clearly in his often-cited prospective study of hope, optimism, and health conducted in 1997 with fifty-seven students, and published in *Psychological Reports*.

At the start of the investigation, Dr. Scioli measured levels of hope and optimism, sorting out surface or self-reported feelings and thoughts, which indicate optimism, versus hope, a deeper emotion revealed through questions designed to identify feelings the respondent might not be conscious of experiencing. The health of each participant was surveyed at both the beginning and end of the study. The more hopeful respondents reported fewer illnesses and rated their illnesses as less severe as compared to those with lower hope scores.

But back to the question, "What's the danger of encouraging someone to look on the bright side?" Doesn't that lead to hope? Doesn't it shine a light on the path to a better future? Numerous studies show that people who think positively are happier, but the problem is, sometimes it's neither possible nor even advisable to be jocular, particularly when you face a disease as grave as cancer.

Some days are lousy, and I can't imagine having to spend those days trying to psych myself out with positive psychobabble. That would take far too much energy and I can't imagine the pressure if I believed a negative thought could cause my cancer to come back.

—R.K., leukemia survivor

"If you believe that your recovery depends on your attitude, then you feel this terrible pressure, like 'How can I be positive when I'm so miserable?'" said journalist and cancer survivor Barbara Ehrenreich. The author of the best seller *Nickel and Dimed*, which highlighted the struggles of low-wage workers, Ehrenreich was now highlighting the lowlights of positive thinking in her new book, best seller *Bright-Sided: How Positive Thinking Is Undermining America*, offering as an alternative, compassion.

The seed for *Bright-Sided* was planted ten years earlier when Ehrenreich, newly diagnosed with breast cancer, got a hefty dose of the "pink ribbon culture's" exhortation to just think positively, which, she writes, "attempts to transform breast cancer into a rite or passage—not an injustice or a tragedy to rail against, but a normal marker in the life cycle, like menopause or grandmotherhood." The seed germinated years later when, while researching a book about white-collar layoffs, she realized those who'd been downsized got the same line as people with cancer.

"I began to see how ubiquitous it is in our culture," she said, and then recited, "This is not a bad thing, this is an opportunity for growth, and renewal, blah blah;" and "you have to think positively to get through it"— because nobody wants to be around anyone negative!

"It's cruel and it's also false," Ehrenreich said.

Dr. Groopman has seen it from the other side of the stethoscope. "It's wrong, it has no scientific basis and it's very, very cruel to the patient," he said, "because you're basically saying you're responsible for your cancer and because you're having negative thoughts or because you're despairing, you're going to be responsible for your own demise."

Indeed. "The failure to think positively can weigh on a patient like a second disease," wrote Ehrenreich.

Psychiatrist Jimmie Holland has seen that happen far too often. She wrote in *The Human Side of Cancer*, about the "Tyranny of Positive Thinking."

"For most patients, cancer is the most difficult and frightening experience they have ever encountered. All this hype claiming that if you don't have a positive attitude and that if you get depressed you are making your tumor grow faster invalidates people's natural and understandable reactions to a threat to their lives.

"This problem has been brought to me by well-meaning families who say, for example, 'You have to help Dad. He's going to die because he isn't positive and he's not trying.' On meeting Dad, I see that he clearly is a stoic, a man who copes well in his own quiet way. Maintaining a positive attitude just isn't his style. Insisting that he put on a happy face and cope in a way that would be foreign to him would actually be an added burden. To rob him of a coping mechanism that has worked before seems unfair. . . ."

David Spiegel, MD, Director of Stanford University's Center on Stress and Health says what he calls "the prison of positive thinking" can make people feel trapped and emotionally constricted. "You know, 'I can only feel good about this, and if I start feeling bad there's something wrong with me,'" he said.

It can also inhibit opportunities for intimacy and emotional interactions. "If you're sitting there crying and your son comes in and says what's the matter, Mom, it can be a moment of real closeness," said Dr. Spiegel. "She says, 'I'm worried that I'm not going to see you get married or go to college'—those can be moments that he will treasure the rest of his life whatever happens. But if you're busy saying, 'Oh, everything's fine dear, I'll be okay,'" you lose opportunities for genuine intimacy that you otherwise would have."

Thinking realistically, or realistic optimism, can provide opportunities for growth and healing, and some maintain that thinking negatively can even be a positive. In *The Positive Power of Negative Thinking*, psychologist Julie K. Norem, PhD, details her scientific research on "defensive pessimism," and tells stories of "people who have harnessed the power of their negative think-ing to increase their self-esteem and make significant progress toward their personal goals." Psychologist Barbara Held, in her book, *Stop Smiling, Start Kvetching: A 5-Step Guide to Creative Complaining*, maintains that com-plaining helps you connect with others and receive support, reorganize your thoughts, and think about your problems in different ways.

Dr. Holland told me that telling a patient to think positively can actu-ally hurt them. "We want people to say when they're depressed and don't feel good—or else we're not going to be able to help them."

Insisting that people who are ill think positively may even endanger their health, because hiding anger or fear can keep you from acknowledging symptoms that warrant attention.

Halina Irving offers a historical perspective. "Over the centuries human beings have dealt with their fear of catastrophe or disease by saying to them-selves, 'This happened to that person because they thought negatively or they led a stressful life.' In past centuries, they said it was because they had unclean thoughts, because they were immoral, because they were witches, because they were bad people.

"I believe that the connotation of 'badness' is attached to so-called neg-ative thinking," continued Irving, "and if you're a good person then you'll think positively, and if you think positively then you have a better chance of getting well. It's blaming the victim."

Irving says we blame the victim because it makes us feel safer. If we assure ourselves that keeping stress at bay will keep the cancer away, we feel like we have control. But this does a great disservice to the patient, says Irving, because now, "not only do they have to suffer the pain of the can-cer, the fear that they're going to die, and the pain of treatment, but also the reality that they will be seen by others in a negative light if they don't get better."

Keep the candle burning

Whenever I write about the admonition "You just have to think positively!" in blog posts, comments flood in. After writing about my interview with Barbara Ehrenreich, one man wrote, "This is one of the toughest subjects that I've dealt with in regard to my cancer struggle. People want to blow rainbows up my rear. . . . If it were a matter of being positive, I'd have been cured the first two times I had treatment for cancer! Now I'm in my third treatment for cancer and I'm still getting the same song and dance from people and it's frustrating."

A newly diagnosed MD wrote: "Even though I know my prognosis is supposed to be good, I find myself feeling so depressed with intermittent crying jags. And of course, everyone says to just 'be positive,' or 'look on the bright side,' especially because they know this type of cancer is usually 'curable.' But I, who am a physician as well, have never been a patient before. Nice to know it's potentially human nature if I can't or don't want to just see the positives in my situation, as a recently diagnosed cancer patient."

A woman wrote about her mother, who was recently diagnosed with ovarian cancer and was terrified that she was hurting her chance of survival because she couldn't seem to get her mind in a positive state. "The irony is that on the few occasions when I could convince my mom to 'just feel' whatever feelings were present and talk about them," wrote the daughter, "she would tell me about her fears, and cry, and then I would watch her whole body relax, and then she would feel more optimistic."

I wrote recently about a study published in the March 2010 *Journal of Thoracic Oncology* that contradicts the older, previously mentioned Australian study about positive thinking's inability to impact lung cancer mortality. The newer study showed that lung cancer patients with an optimistic attitude survived an average of six months longer compared to their pessimistic counterparts. This hit a hot button with many readers, but some readers were more sanguine:

> *I am not a "power of positive thinking" person. I am a complex human being with intricately woven responses to optimism, pessimism, hope, fear, faith, and G-d. I detest when people tell me that I have to think optimistically.*
>
> —D.B., breast cancer survivor

"I don't think staying positive means you go through an ordeal (cancer or otherwise) with a constant smile on your face and a string of 'don't worry, be happy' quotes; sometimes being positive, in the midst of incredible odds against you, is just a willingness to get out of bed, brush your teeth, comb your hair (if you didn't lose it all!) and face the day that awaits you."

Hope killers

So if telling people they have to think positively or have hope can actually harm them, what can friends and loved ones do to inspire hope, without exactly saying so? First, consider the most common hope killers.

"One is the view of illness as punishment," said Dr. Groopman. "You know, 'This is happening to me because I did something wrong,' and in a religious framework that can happen because of a distorted theology."

And although suggesting that your friend think positively can have the opposite effect, you can keep it positive by refraining from sharing bad news about the world, news that could instill fear and anxiety, cast out hope, and trigger an adrenaline-powered fight-or-flight reaction.

It was difficult for me to hear from my husband that I need to stop feeling sorry for myself at times when I was depressed or needed to cry.

—M.M., breast cancer survivor

You can read more about keeping hope alive in part II, but here's an easy-to-remember tip: To foster *hope*, encourage *humor* when appropriate, and no cancer *horror* stories, ever.

As the revised edition of this book goes to press, Joanne remains well and happy. It's been eleven years since her doctor told her she had six months to live.

I wouldn't be bold enough to say that hope has kept her alive. But I can say with utter impunity that hope has helped her live a better life. And the example of her spirit and drive has given me and countless others, including her doctor, immeasurable hope.

9.

"I want you to respect my judgment and treatment decisions."

To be trusted is a greater compliment than being loved.

—George MacDonald

"I SHOULD HAVE CALLED YOU MONTHS AGO," I chided myself silently as her blue eyes tracked me from the hospital room doorway to her bedside.

"Hi, Lori," said Roxanne, smiling and dimpling her cheek. I planted a kiss on it and gave her a hug.

"So what's going on?" I pulled up a chair so we would be at eye level, something I learned from *Give Me Your Hand*, a Jewish healing guide to visiting the ill.

"I'd been bleeding for a long time," she began. "I thought it was menopause, crazy periods, and I was so busy taking care of Dad, plus work has been insane. . . ." A loud sigh. "So this morning I was really bleeding, I mean *really*. My assistant brought me to the ER. I have cervical cancer."

"Didn't you get pap smears?" I asked—but again, silently, catching myself before the words arrowed their way to her heart.

"Oh, Rox. I am so sorry."

I was sorry not only for her diagnosis, which I knew something about, having received a similarly terrifying diagnosis three years earlier, but also for all she'd been through with her dad, who had been living with her for almost a year.

"Dad was getting impossible to take care of," she said. "He was almost blind, and I had to do personal care things that, well, I can't even talk about. Then I had to find him a home and get him moved, all the while I was selling houses and working all hours."

"Why didn't you call me?" I asked, knowing that Rox was not one to complain, confide, or request help, and feeling more contrite that I had not checked in with her for so long.

"I knew how busy you were. And I've been totally exhausted."

It was 2005, the height of the real estate boom, and Rox had finally realized her lifelong dream of financial success. But it came at a steep cost; she worked in a high-stress business with blurred work-life boundaries. Reminded me of my life as a documentary producer. But Roxanne, without siblings, a mate, children, or able-bodied parents, was on her own. She did have friends, but some, like me, had stepped back after not hearing from her for so long. I had taken it personally, and thought that because she didn't return a couple of my calls, she didn't really care about me.

But now, this could not be *about me*. It had to be about her, this stoic, statuesque blonde with a fierce Protestant work ethic who was certainly not Protestant. As I would learn, she was a Christian Scientist, which explained why she didn't get pap smears.

How could I not be aware of that when I'd known her for seven years? Because we were not intimates. We were neighbors first—she moved in two doors up, immigrating to our relatively suburban Oakland neighborhood from San Francisco—and our friendship was rooted in barbeques, yard sales, and shared Meyer lemons. We also shared an intellectual curiosity, but our belief systems stood worlds apart. After we attended a seminar together with Wayne Dyer, author of *The Power of Intention: Change Your Mind, Change Your Life*, I questioned some of his assertions, positing that although I believe your thoughts shape your reality, there are some realities so strong that they persist no matter what. "It's all in your mind," Rox said emphatically. We argued amicably, but endlessly: an unlikely and emotion-

---

Not helpful: "Maybe you should stop drinking diet pop and try these special vitamins that worked for my cousin Irving's prostate."

—B.C. breast cancer survivor

ally distant pair that never took our differences too seriously and always found something to joke about. After seeing Mr. Dyer, we subsequently referred to him as "D-wayne D-wyer."

Never did Roxanne reveal to me the sad or dark hollows of her soul. I thought it was because she was so private, but soon realized that she withheld complaint because she believed that by acknowledging negative feelings she gave them dominion. This was the belief of a woman raised in the Christian Science faith, who later become a staunch follower of the dogma of intentionality.

Before Roxanne's cancer, I had no idea that she eschewed conventional medicine. Nor did I realize that once she was hospitalized in an emergency situation, she would deem it permissible to accept conventional treatment. That never quite made sense to me. But that was just the beginning of a long vexation with things I may never understand.

Rox was hospitalized for almost a month. Her grapefruit-sized tumor sustained almost daily doses of radiation. Eager to give back for all Rox had done for my family and me when I had cancer—she was an attentive and generous friend—and perhaps motivated by guilt over letting our friendship lapse without considering what she was going through—I decided I would be there for her, unconditionally. During her hospitalization, I visited frequently. At her behest, I shared the news of her cancer with her friends and neighbors, and helped create a community of care to support her at home during her six weeks of chemo when she needed rides, meals, housekeeping help, and more than anything, love and acceptance.

⌐⌐⌐

"You're cured," declared the square-jawed surgeon from behind his massive desk, rocking side to side in triumph. A few days earlier Rox had undergone a biopsy to learn the results of the radiation and chemo. A smile electrified her face.

"There's no evidence of cancer," he continued. "So there's nothing else to do. No need for a hysterectomy—your body has had enough trauma, anyway—so just go home, enjoy your life, and come back to see me in three months."

Words and thoughts indeed shape our perceptions, even when we know the words may be at worst, false and, at best, misleading. How could Roxanne's tumor and any residual cells have been totally obliterated? It mattered not: we both believed in miracles, and more important, wanted to believe what we heard. So we did. And for the rest of the summer we delighted in every normal, mundane moment.

But those would be the last normal moments of Rox's life. The next biopsy revealed cancerous cells that the surgeon said had certainly spread beyond her uterus.

"But you said I was *cured*," Roxanne protested.

"There was no evidence of disease, so you *were* cured," replied the surgeon.

I felt the blood drain from my face as if I was hearing that *my* cancer had returned. First devastated, then furious, then panicked, I tried to keep a calm and confident face.

I still don't know whether to love or hate that surgeon for the reprieve he gave us, and I still wonder whether I could have softened the blow by warning Roxanne earlier that he could have meant something other than "cured" when he used that word. Today I would ask for an explanation from the surgeon, though not in Roxanne's presence. I now prefer the term, NED or "No evidence of disease" to "cure," because, truly, no one can ever truly know whether they're cured. (See chapter 20.)

Roxanne could not tolerate more radiation, not even radiation seeds, according to the radiologists we consulted. She could have undergone more chemotherapy, but it would buy a few months at best, so we investigated complementary therapies. A friend told me about an acupuncturist and Chinese herbalist who conducted a study at Stanford University showing the therapeutic value of a certain kind of mushroom, so in the leaf-stripping rains of autumn, we drove to San Francisco where Roxanne lay in a dark room with fine needles carefully placed at multiple meridians, and then found our way to a deep, narrow shop in Chinatown where we paid more than a hundred dollars for a bag of dried mushrooms to brew into a healing tea.

Roxanne downed the foul-tasting stuff for many weeks without complaint. But one day when I asked about the acupuncture and mushrooms, she said, "I'm not doing that anymore. I'm just going on with my life."

I wanted to argue with her, but what could I say? I had researched clinical trials, and found no matches. She felt fine, she said, and wanted to get back to work, not in real estate—too demanding—but in something else.

We continued to get together often and for me, life got back to normal. Rox seemed her old cheerful, wry, fun-loving self. She came over often and we'd perch at our breakfast bar and chat, or take in lectures at the Commonwealth Club in San Francisco. Life went on like that until mid-July, when Rox called one afternoon and asked if I could give her a hand with dinner. She said she'd pulled a muscle in her back and had ordered grocery deliveries from Safeway for a few days but now had a tough time getting to the kitchen.

"Have you called the doctor?" I asked.

"I know what he'll say. 'Just rest and you'll be fine.'"

"But maybe he could prescribe some meds," I insisted.

"Naw," she said. "I'm not going to the doctor."

"How about I call the advice nurse and just to see. It couldn't hurt."

"Lori. NO."

"But. . ."

"Listen, if you'd rather not come over that's okay—I'll be fine."

My mom died of breast cancer at twenty-eight. I fought to have a complete mastectomy rather than the then-popular lumpectomies. I was blatantly accused of craziness and self-mutilation by friends, coworkers, and my lover at the time. I was shunned rather than supported. I am alive ten years later and my kids have a mom against overwhelming odds.

—L.H. breast cancer survivor

That was that. So began two weeks of almost daily visits, in which I delighted in the warm glow of Roxanne's sunlit living room, painted pale butter yellow. Rox had spent the past two years decorating her home just to her liking, and now we got to sit and enjoy it uninterrupted and with impunity during the long days of summer. Rox kept her feet up on the sofa and her legs stretched out—otherwise she became uncomfortable—so I served her dinner on a tray that she placed on her lap.

I suspected that her cancer had returned, and continued suggesting pain medication or a doctor's visit. But she was intransigent.

I wish I had been able to derive some satisfaction when she finally asked me to take her to the hospital. It was a Saturday night in early August, and David and I were on our way to dinner, when my cell phone rang.

"How you doin,' Rox?"

"I need to go to the emergency room."

She was bleeding again.

"Oh, Rox," I said as we waited in the ER for what felt like hours. "Why didn't you tell me?"

"What could you have done? I'm working on this, Lori. For a long time, I've been working with a Christian Science practitioner on my healing, on getting my mind right. I'm going to get well. I just have to work on getting my mind right."

She had been bleeding for months, but hadn't told a soul except her healer, whom I had no idea existed and who told Roxanne that neither her pain nor her cancer were real.

Part of me felt grateful that Rox had finally confided in me, but another part fumed. If she had let me take her to the doctor earlier I would not be sharing her pain and staying up all night with her. But how could I feel angry at a woman bone tired and suffering, a friend whom I loved in spite of how virulently I disagreed with her? It was impossible to change her. I could choose compassion. Or I could choose to leave.

The cancer was back. She agreed to an oncologist visit, but she said that she didn't want to hear anything about the tumor because it would impair the healing she was working on with her practitioner. So she asked me to see him as her medical proxy. While she read a magazine in the waiting room, I faced the reality she chose to ignore.

"Where's the patient?" asked the oncologist. I explained that she was a Christian Scientist and did not want to hear about cancer.

"But she should know this," he said.

"She knows what she needs to know," I said, holding back tears. "This is her religion. She doesn't want to know. She wants me to know because she respects my reality, like I respect hers."

Clearly annoyed, he rolled his eyes and proceeded to show me the CT scan on his computer monitor as if it he was explaining a weather map. It revealed a storm, a hurricane of cancer.

"I can approve hospice care," he said.

"It's bad, Rox," I said, taking her hand from her lap. I persuaded her to walk to the hospice office with me since it was just a block away. We met

> *I had a long talk with a friend who is a homeopathic practitioner. He kept encouraging me to deny chemo, that it was poison. It didn't help me at all. My choice wasn't respected, and I was left with a sinking suspicion that I may be choosing to poison myself.*
>
> —T.A., stomach cancer survivor

with the director and Rox seemed open to receiving hospice care, but said she wanted to think about it.

The next afternoon her living room was strangely brighter than it had ever been before.

"I don't want hospice now. And I don't want people to know this time," she said.

"I understand," I said, "You don't want people to treat you differently," thinking of one of the statements that people with cancer said in my first survivor survey that they want others to know, "I want to be treated kindly, not differently."

"No, that's not it. I don't want them to think of me as sick because that will keep me sick. How people think of you affects who you are."

"That's ridiculous," I thought, but knew by then that what I believed was of no consequence and could only undermine her healing. Her one hope for a cure lay in her ability to shape her reality through her thoughts.

The next three months were among the most demanding, sad, and perhaps most enriching of my life. As Roxanne grew sicker, our community of care grew smaller. She hired a part-time caregiver and refused to see most of her friends because it took too much energy, energy she wanted to save for her healing work. I think she let me into her world because I not only accepted her choices, but also demanded so little of her. Sometimes we would simply be together, wordless, she in her bed, I on the loveseat. She would nap. I would read.

I occasionally brought up hospice. "You don't have to die once you're admitted. Some people leave hospice care without dying. And that's okay."

But she refused.

I wish I could say I continued to be the loving and accepting friend I fancied myself. But I could see the pain on Roxanne's face, and it worsened, in spite of her Christian Science reading and counseling. She had been taking Vicodin occasionally, even though her "healer" discouraged that, but it wasn't working well enough, and I couldn't bear to see Roxanne suffer. I called her oncologist's nurse to see what else we might try.

"I'm not a pain specialist," she said. "That's what hospice nurses do, manage pain. You need to get Roxanne into hospice."

"But she refuses," I said. "What am I supposed to do?"

"Well, let me ask you this: what are you going to do when she dies?"

"I don't know. Call 911, I guess."

"No, that's not what you want to do," she said. "If there's any kind of problem, you could be implicated, legally. If she's in hospice care, they take care of all of that. You call them and they know exactly what to do."

It felt like emotional blackmail or praying when I kneeled by Roxanne's bed, where she had stayed for almost two weeks.

"Rox, I don't know what to do. I'm trying to get you some different meds to help you, and the oncology nurse just told me that if you're not in hospice and something happens. . . ." I could not bring myself to say it at first, but then it came: "If you die, I could get in trouble."

That was all it took. "Okay, my Lori," she sighed.

Within a day, a hospice social worker and a nurse visited. Roxanne still resisted pain medications—her Christian Science practitioner kept telling her she needed to get her mind right and she'd be fine—but toward the end, she relented.

The afternoon before Rox died, I sat at her bed and we exchanged a very long, expressive, loving look. Then she gave me a sweet dimpled smile.

"Lori, there is so much I want to tell you. But I'm so tired."

"It's okay. I hear you. I love you."

"I love you, Lori."

⧉⧉⧉

Respecting Roxanne's judgment and palliative care decisions challenged and changed me in ways I never could have imagined. Her choices—and mine—haunt me to this day. Could I have been more insistent, forceful even? Certainly. But the truth is, had I been, she would not have accepted my presence, my compassion, and perhaps my love.

Worse, the sadness and fear that she died blaming herself for not being able to "get her mind right" will forever dog me.

Speaking at Roxanne's memorial in the vaulted-ceiling living room of a neighbor, I tried to explain to the friends who were ignorant about her recurrence why she didn't want any but her closest friends to know. I'm not sure everyone understood. But it didn't matter. I loved Roxanne well. And together we proved that love is stronger than thought. Love creates its own reality. Love somehow miraculously heals everyone in its midst.

Reconciling what you think you know with what the person with cancer wants

Like me, Dr. Jeff Kane, also a student of philosophy, sometimes raises tough, knotty questions. About the statement, "I want you to respect my judgment and treatment decisions," he asked, "As helpers (a relative, say, or even group facilitator), how do I feel when the person with cancer decides on a course I think is absolutely nuts or even potentially harmful? At that point, the suffering might be *mine*, so how do I address that?"

To quote the Serenity Prayer, as Dr. Marty Rossman does in describing the foundation of the program he outlines in *The Worry Solution*: "Lord, grant me the serenity to accept those things I cannot change, the courage to change the things I can change, and the wisdom to know the difference."

Dr. Rossman believes that we have more wisdom within us than we use. "This is especially true," he wrote, "when we are anxious, stressed, or worried, because fear tends to cause a psychological phenomenon called regression." This makes our thinking more childlike, possibly precluding our ability to access our adult wisdom.

This holds true not just for cancer survivors, but also their friends and loved ones. When we hear that someone we love has cancer, we fear not only for him or her, but also usually for ourselves. We may fear losing our beloved or the life we share with them. We may worry we could fall prey to the same disease. So how do we find the "wisdom to know the difference" between the support our loved may say she needs and the medical support we believe she actually needs, keeping in mind that it gets to be about our loved one now, not us?

Recently cancer survivor, author, speaker and physician Wendy Harpham, MD, wrote a series of posts on her Healthy Survivor blog regarding patients' belief in the power of positive thinking. She asked readers, at the end of one post, "Is it wrong to hold your tongue and let them believe what they want to believe while they are still doing well?"

> *I made it very clear that I am doing the best I can under the circumstances and I will not accept any discussions about things that cannot be undone or changed, and that are not helping me in any way.*
>
> —A.R. breast cancer survivor

I answered, "I believe that disabusing patients' belief in the power of positive thinking is wrong, not because I believe in the power of positive thinking to heal or cure, but because I believe in supporting the faith and belief of anyone rendered raw, vulnerable, and traumatized by disease. 'Whatever gets you through the night,' I say—just so it's not hurting someone else."

But what if patients are hurting themselves, as Roxanne was? Dr. Harpham followed up on this issue, reframing the question.

"Do you say something? Do you forcibly drag your friend in to see a doctor? Are you your friend's keeper? Your intent may be wholesome, but there are boundaries around what you can say and do. Assuming your friend is not psychotic or unconscious (in which case, call 911), here are some thoughts."

She quoted from her book, *When a Parent Has Cancer*:

"[Y]ou can't make the decisions or take charge of the problems. . . . Premise all your words and actions on your belief that . . . you respect their right to choose how they handle *their* crisis. Make it clear . . . they are in control of how much you help, and that you will respect their wishes. . . .

"Stay alert for windows of opportunity to mention your concerns. Unless . . . [they] ask you not to bring up the topic, try again and again. . . .

"When the chemistry simply isn't good for sharing your thoughts . . . try getting the information to the . . . [patients] through one of their close friends, clergy, or someone else they trust and respect. . . .

"Ultimately, it is their life and they have a right to live it their way. Recognizing and respecting your limits in their lives is one of the ultimate expressions of love."

And one of the most challenging ones.

10.

"I want you to give me an opening to talk about cancer, and then take my lead."

It is only with the heart that one can see rightly:
What is essential is invisible to the eye.

—Antoine de Saint-Exupéry

"SO HOW ARE YOU?" asked Jessie at a barbeque under a canopy of a massive redwood that shaded most of her back yard.

"I'm doing great," enthused Tammy. She was in the midst of chemo, which explained why a wig had transformed her from a brunette to a redhead. "How's everything with you?"

"No, I mean, how are you *doing*?"

"Wonderfully, thanks," replied Tammy. "What a day, huh? Can't wait to bite into that chicken—smells delish!"

"Can you eat okay? I mean, aren't you nauseated from chemo?"

"I'm having a great day! So how's your family," asked Tammy, trying again to deflect the conversation away from herself.

"Everybody's healthy! How's your daughter taking your cancer?"

Jessie may have been denser than the redwood tree she stood under. Although Tammy let her know in so many words—and certainly more than enough words—that she wasn't in the mood for cancer-chat, Jessie just couldn't or wouldn't get it.

"The big message is that the healthy person interacting with the sick person must learn how to take communicative lead," said Lisa Sparks, whose fifty-eight-year-old father died of lung cancer when she was a graduate student. Now with a PhD in communications, Dr. Sparks teaches at the Comprehensive Cancer Center at University of California, Irvine, taking an evidence-based approach to bring about health behavior change.

I asked Dr. Sparks what "taking the communicative lead" means.

"You listen. You shut up and listen!" she exclaimed.

That often means waiting for the cancer combatant to bring up the subject of health instead of introducing it yourself. Once the conversation about cancer has begun, however, Dr. Sparks said we can practice communication techniques shown to smooth rather than ruffle feathers. Saying things like "It's not fair," makes the patient feel less responsible for his or her illness.

Some days, I didn't want to hear anything about cancer. I wanted friends and others to let me lead that part of the conversation. And I'm still not a huge fan of detailed stories of people who thought they'd recovered, only to have a recurrence years later.

—D.C., breast cancer survivor

"That's what we call 'equivocal communication,' sort of a neutralizing message. That's a good strategy. It doesn't always work, but it's a good starting point."

Sparks said the most important principle of communication is audience analysis. Who are you dealing with? She gave an example.

"One of my colleagues has cancer right now," she began. "He was diagnosed with colorectal cancer six months ago. So, of course, I know all the literature. I could be a 'know it all,' of course, but I'm not. And I just have to remember my audience."

A private person, Sparks's colleague did not want to talk about his cancer, but loved talking about his teaching and goings-on within his department. He also loved junk food and drinking.

"So I leave all these funny messages on his machine, just randomly, I'll say, 'Hey, I'm at Burger King. If you're having a bad day and don't feel like cooking, this place is fantastic!' And I leave these messages just trying to make him laugh. And then I gave him a bottle of port, because I know he likes it and he survived his chemotherapy round. Anyone who can survive that deserves to celebrate."

Finally, Dr. Sparks added, "And when I talk to him, I don't ever bring up the cancer. And if he brings it up, I listen. I shut up and listen."

Dr. Sparks thought it was easier for her colleague to spend time with her than others because she does not judge or attempt to control him.

"You'd think I'd be saying, 'Read this, read that, here's this article,' but I don't do any of that. Because of that, I think he respects me even more as a human being, knowing that I'm just a friend."

By watching and listening to her colleague, Dr. Sparks has learned what he wants and needs.

> *I just wanted it to be normal. My friend came and we played Scrabble and talked, and it helped. Sometimes we talked about cancer. Sometimes we did not. But we played Scrabble just as we had for most of our friendship.*
>
> —A.T., breast cancer survivor

It's not just what you say or how you say it

Actions can indeed speak louder than words. Up to three-quarters of human communication takes place nonverbally. Thankfully, we can learn to better read face and body language.

Psychology professor and renowned nonverbal communication expert Paul Ekman, PhD, wrote the book, so to speak, on facial expressions. His classic, *Telling Lies*, which studies the hundreds of facial muscles and expressions that reveal whether we are telling the truth or not, was the basis for the Emmy-winning television crime drama television series *Lie to Me*, seen in more than fourteen countries.

Dr. Ekman says we can learn to recognize genuine emotions, and even "microexpressions," which he defines as "very fast facial movements lasting less than one-fifth of a second [that] are an important source of leakage," meaning that they can reveal an emotion a person is trying to conceal.

"If you read it in their face," Dr. Ekman said, "then you should resonate with the emotion they're feeling to show you not only recognize it but you feel it to some extent."

Although it can help to read someone's face and know what they are feeling and reverberate that, it's more complicated than that.

"Emotions never tell you their cause. When you see anger in a patient, you don't know if it's anger about being sick or the fact that her friends are abandoning her or the fact that the nurse didn't show up for thirty minutes. You have to find that out, and say, 'You're upset; it looks like something's driving you nuts, and we need to talk about it.'"

But Dr. Ekman adds that it's not always safe to be so direct. "When I saw a microexpression on a friend's face when I was visiting him after he had open heart surgery, the most I would say is 'Everything okay? Anything you want to talk about?' because if it is a microexpression, they're either unaware of how they're feeling or they're very much aware of it but they're trying to conceal it, so you have to handle that with delicacy."

Sometimes, even if you're well-versed in facial and body language, even if you have a high Emotional Intelligence Quotient (EIQ), it can be impossible to know what a person with cancer wants or needs. While it would be pretty obvious to most what Tammy needed at the party, it's not always so simple. Some may resent it if you don't ask after their health, particularly when they're in the throes of treatment.

"I didn't want to upset you," said Alan to his friend, Lily, who had finally confronted him weeks after she was diagnosed about why he never asked how she was feeling.

"Honesty is the best policy." Trite. But true. When I feel unable to read another person, which is common when you're on the phone, and nigh impossible when you're communicating via email, unless you have a very wide range of emoticons at your disposal, I simply ask.

"I'm not sure whether to ask about your health because you may not want to talk about it," I might say. "Would you like me to bring it up? Or would you rather be the one to bring it up? I hope I'm not upsetting you by mentioning it now."

By pulling the protective sheet off the elephant in the room, revealing its massive body, you may more easily move the pachyderm elsewhere.

Again, keep it about the person who has cancer; step outside yourself and put yourself not just in their shoes, but also in their very heart. Listen. Learn. Love. And then act accordingly.

11.

"I want compassion, not pity."

To be unhappy is only half the misfortune—
to be pitied—is misery complete.

—Arthur Schnitzler

I DON'T REMEMBER HOW OLD I WAS when I first discovered what made me feel freakishly different from everyone else. But I do remember feeling hideous and branded. Fortunately, I was able to hide my birthmarks beneath my clothing, and as a young woman, have them surgically removed. But the shame had taken root and ran so deep that I didn't feel I could share my secret with anyone. It seems so silly now.

But if I realize how silly it was, why haven't I told anyone?

Humans are the most social of animals. In our earliest day as *Australopithecus*, if we didn't fit into the group and were banished, we would die. As one prostate cancer said, he didn't tell anyone he had cancer because he didn't want to be "cut off from the herd."

We do not want to be alone and we do not want to *feel* alone. (This is not to say we don't enjoy solitude, which implies choice. But that's a different conversation.) That was why my birthmarks—button-sized supernumerary nipples just beneath my breasts—aroused such fear that I would be ridiculed and ostracized if anyone knew. I felt cursed, and carried the lonely burden through my childhood and adolescence, until a surgeon replaced the nipples with two short scars. Even years later, shame bloomed on my face when I heard the joke, "Martinis are like a woman's breasts: one's not enough and three's too many."

Thirty years later, being diagnosed with lung cancer was the closest I had come since then to experiencing such isolation, fear, and shame. I had smoked in my youth, and although my oldest friends knew that, most who knew me for less than two decades had no idea. Almost every time I shared my diagnosis, unwitting colleagues and acquaintances gasped, "But you never smoked!" Sheepishly, I would admit, "Yes I did. But I quit almost twenty years ago."

Sometimes I saw judgment in their eyes. Other times I simply felt alone. But when people said, "I used to smoke, too," I felt a sameness, a sense of compassion, like they knew that they could be in the same boat, as anyone could be and indeed as we all are. As Buddhist nun Pema Chödrön said, "Life is getting on a boat going out to sea that is going to sink."

Psychiatrist Jimmie Holland pointed out in *The Human Side of Cancer*, "It makes no sense to blame the person who is ill. Being ill makes one feel alone enough, and being blamed adds to a feeling of distance and isolation, of somehow being 'different' from others in a way we've never experienced before."

We all need to feel a sense of sameness and camaraderie.

And compassion.

Compassion defined

Chödrön wrote in *The Places That Scare You: A Guide to Fearlessness in Difficult Times*, "Compassion is not a relationship between the healer and the wounded. It's a relationship between equals . . . [it] becomes real when we recognize our shared humanity."

The prefix "com" in compassion means "with or together," as in "combine." Partnered with "passion," *compassion* means to "feel" with.

Although compassion is often used as a synonym for "pity" in dictionaries, I see them and their distinct effects as vastly different. I met a man of great compassion who agreed, and explained why.

Compassion vs. pity

It was 6:30 a.m. and still dark in the high-ceilinged industrial kitchen of the Santa Sabina Retreat Center in Marin County, California, where I was taking a private writing retreat. Groggy, I turned the corner from the stainless steel table in the middle of the kitchen and shuffled into the narrow pantry, where refrigerators and freezers buzzed. My heart jumped; a man in a green flannel robe stood inches away and a foot above me. His happy black eyes immediately assuaged my fear.

"Good morning!" he whispered loudly.

Though we likely hailed from different universes, I took an immediate liking to this bear of a man, and was surprised to learn after a few minutes of small talk that he was a priest who had traveled across the country from North Carolina to lead the Easter Retreat that would start later that day.

I told him I was a writer working on a book about how to best support people with cancer, and he nodded knowingly. We chatted for a few minutes about well-meaning friends and family, and it became apparent that, even though he had never suffered from cancer, he had yearned for compassion.

As we were about to part, coffee cups in hand, we realized we had not exchanged names. "I'm Jude Siciliano," he said.

The next day I awakened, again predawn, with a compulsion to ask this man of the cloth about the difference between compassion and pity. I ran downstairs to look for him, and there he stood, just outside the kitchen.

"I've been thinking about the difference between pity and compassion, and for some reason I think you have something to say about that."

"I do," he smiled. We walked through the glass doors to the grassy rear courtyard and sat at a picnic table. I turned on my tape recorder, and as he spoke, I watched this warm man in sweats and slippers morph into an erudite scholar.

"When I do reflections with people in scripture groups and people have a chance to reflect on their reactions," he began, "one of the words they take offense at is the word 'pity'—like 'Jesus having pity'—and it's used a lot in the New Testament. But it's an Old Testament term, too.

"In the New Testament, Jesus has pity on people who are diseased or in need, as in 'Jesus had pity on him and he reached out and touched the man and the man could see.' But people in groups say, 'I don't like the word pity because it sounds condescending, and who wants pity?'

It was such a scary period of my life. I sometimes felt like I had to be strong and keep up a good face, because I didn't want people to feel sorry for me. At times, I wish I could've let others know how bad I really felt.

—D.N., endometrial cancer survivor

"Pity is what you do when you toss some money to someone in the street," Father Siciliano continued. "Somehow there's this feeling of aboveness."

A better translation of the word that is used in the Bible is "compassion," he explained. "The Greek word is 'compassion' and it means a feeling that comes from the womb or the bowels. It's what a parent feels when a child falls and cries—that instinctual feeling that arises for something you want to respond to. A woman once told me when her child falls and she hears it crying, the milk in her breast flows. That's physical and emotional."

He then explained the Latin origin of "compassion," which means to "suffer with." "So that's different from having pity and looking down on someone as if you're the physician and they're the sick person; you're the one above looking at them below.

"Compassion is when you feel the pain but don't come up with easy answers. It's what I'd want, someone to feel the pain with me, sit with me and not come up with easy answers."

Commiseration

Talia's best friend Zooey offered easy answers when Talia was diagnosed with a rare, treatment-resistant cancer.

An art curator in New York City who jogged five miles the day she was diagnosed, Talia had come to expect success. But when she learned that a year and a half is considered a long survival time for her disease, she realized she might not see her teenage son complete his first year of college. (Thankfully, she did.)

"People think I'll be fine, and they say so," she told me over the phone. "It really upsets me, even when other survivors say that. How the hell do you know?"

It upset her even more when Zooey tried to reassure her.

"She seems to think part of being a friend is thinking it'll be okay. If she would just commiserate, it would help. Don't fix or deny my pain. Just let me feel it," Talia said.

Allowing someone to feel their pain, and feeling their pain with them, can seem dangerous, like running into a burning building. But as Dr. Jeff Kane emphasized, you don't have to let someone else's pain damage you. You can experience it and then let it go. Some caregivers and friends cannot release the pain they have taken in because they want to *control* it—make it go away. That's simply not possible most of the time, but even though you cannot control it, you can make it more bearable by simply opening yourself up and allowing yourself to imagine what the other person is experiencing.

Compassion involves not just feeling with someone, but realizing that you could be going through the same thing—if not the same disease, then the same feeling of imminent disaster, pain, or even death. Compassion leaves no room for judgment or condescension.

Merriam-Webster defines condescension as "voluntary descent from one's rank or dignity in relations with an inferior." But I heard another definition that makes more sense to me: "Condescension is when someone is better off than you and they know it."

Nancy, a friend who offered my husband and me her country cabin when I was recovering from cancer, shared a story she heard from her boss about a woman who was diagnosed with breast cancer at age thirty-four.

"A clueless visitor to the house looked over at the girl in bed and said, 'Thank goodness I always ate a healthy diet and got plenty of exercise. This could never happen to me.'"

Nancy continued, "I don't think there's always a reason why bad things happen. 'Why me?' might as well be 'Why not'?"

Many words of heartfelt compassion without being condescending were said, "I love you" meant a lot to hear, or "You mean so much to me."

—L.C., invasive ductal carcinoma

Do you know how I feel? No.

As important as it is to attempt to put yourself in someone else's shoes and feel compassion, it's just as vital that you keep from diminishing a survivor's experience by saying you know how they feel. Again and again in my survey, survivors commented that they disliked it when people said, "I know how you feel." A breast cancer survivor told a story about this.

"A coworker came in to my office to express sympathy, and then proceeded to tell me he was tested for AIDS and the results were negative. But the person said he knows how I feel because of the fear factor." She didn't share how she felt with her colleague because she knew he meant no harm, but she nonetheless felt disappointed, minimized, sad, and resentful. A man with renal cell carcinoma wrote, "Oftentimes people say 'I know how you feel.' No they do not . . . they do not have cancer." It makes him feel minimized, confused, angry, and sad.

I think no matter how strong a person may try to show they are, they always need a little compassion.

—C.C., early stage breast cancer

When I recently corresponded with a woman whose son died of cancer, I wrote back to her, "I am truly sorry for your loss. I can't understand what it is like to have been through what you have been through and continue to go through, but I can try to imagine it." I then shared that my father had recently died of cancer and how much I missed him, and that although I knew it was nothing like the loss of a child, it was all that I knew at that point."

She wrote back, "I just told my daughter that what you said about missing your dad and how it isn't the same as missing a child, but that it's all you know. [It's] probably one of the nicest, and most appropriate, things anyone has said to me. I think even if someone tried to compare my loss to them losing their dog (which sadly has happened to me), it would be okay if they would just add 'It's all I know' to the end of the statement!"

All we can truly know is that which we have experienced. But we can begin to know if we don't just try to imagine what someone is going through, but take the time to consciously focus on his or her plight. This is why media can be so powerful. After the 2011 earthquake, tsunami, and nuclear reactor cataclysm in Japan, we not only saw the physical ravages, but the internal devastation and horror on the faces of our fellow humans. The cover of

Time magazine showed a close-up of a woman in tears, face like a rumpled rag, her head bowed against a pale lavender towel. How could one help but feel with her?

With cancer, the internal disaster and devastation is less apparent, and sometimes invisible to the eye. Hence the surprise, "But you look so good!" reaction fielded by cancer survivors whose bodies belie the real and true anguish they feel. Though I have no idea what it feels like to be victimized by a titanic natural disaster, and would never presume to know, I do know what having cancer is like. For many of us, the internal implosion feels like an earthquake that cannot be seen; the flood of fear threatens to drown us; the volatility of our emotions feels like a reactor threatening a meltdown.

When you see someone with cancer, look beneath and beyond. And then send love and prayers and good thoughts and hope for healing. And as you thank God or goodness that it is not you, realize that it could be you, and that if it ever is, your friend will certainly be there for you just as you were for her.

12.

"Advice may not be what I need, and it may hurt more than help. Try comforting me instead."

From a good teacher you may learn the secret of listening. You will never learn the secret of life. You will have to listen for yourself.

—Rachel Naomi Remen, MD

MONICA WALKED INTO HER DOCTOR'S OFFICE with "a list of weird symptoms"—night sweats, stopped-up ears, a lump on the left side of her rib cage, and a persistent cough. The doctor irrigated her ears and ordered a CT scan and an ultrasound. Although she told him she thought it was menopause, "I had a sneaking suspicion something was seriously wrong," she said. "I just knew on some level, and I actually made peace with the idea I might have cancer and I might die."

Monica wasn't going to die. She had a highly treatable case of non-Hodgkin's lymphoma. She would, however, need chemotherapy.

Single and fiercely independent, Monica knew what she wanted: to live, and to do so the way *she* wanted. Although she accepted help with certain chores, she wanted to maintain control, as she always had, over what she ate.

"I'm a picky eater anyway, and my sister and friends would shop for me. I'd make a very specific list—'I want Campbell's Bean with Bacon soup.' They'd either come back with the generic brand or give me flak about my food preferences. 'If I want to eat Hostess Twinkies, well, if it will get me through cancer, I'll eat them!' I would say. I had a friend with cancer who had been avoiding nitrites her whole life, and she said, 'I have cancer now so let's have some bacon!'"

People gave Monica printouts about various risk factors and even her five-year survival rate. She threw it all in the recycling bin. "I didn't want that information."

It has been three years since Monica's diagnosis. "When I get to five years, I'll be considered 'cured,'" she laughed. "So I'm going to have a party and serve only cured foods—olives and ham and the like!"

Advice separates

When people we love face a challenge, most of us automatically spring to their aid. Advice is a natural and easy way to help. But any kind of advice, sound or not, can be more hurtful than helpful, especially if we don't fully understand what the person is going through.

"I don't believe in advice, whether we're sick or not, without first asking permission to give advice," said therapist Halina Irving, who is also a support group leader. "I believe that as important as human connections are, our autonomy—our entitlement to our own thoughts and feelings and judgment—is also crucially important." It's even more crucial when people are striving to maintain their dignity, independence, and sense of control in a world that may suddenly feel unmanageable.

Irving said some people want to give advice because they like the superior position of knowing something, which makes the recipient of the advice feel put down. "But some people want to give advice because they really think they have something of value to impart," she added. Even so, they should first ask, saying something like, "I have some thoughts about what you're going through. Would you like to hear them? My feelings will not be hurt if you'd rather not hear it."

"You just need to stay positive and remember all that has been given to you," [said] a church leader and a best friend. I was in the hospital, literally fighting for my life with complications from surgery. Because I tend to be a pleaser, I smiled and agreed. Yet, another reason for why it hurt so much. I was angry with myself, too.

—T.L., invasive lobular carcinoma survivor

Irving said, as a cancer patient, it's easier to accept advice from someone who has had cancer, but in her support groups she emphasizes that the group's goal is not to advise. "This is about sharing our own experiences," she tells members, "and as you express your own experience, someone else might find something useful in it, something that we haven't thought of."

Just because someone has had cancer doesn't mean what worked for them will work for someone else. Soon after I was diagnosed, I was offered advice by a lung cancer survivor I'll call Paul whose words left me thunderstruck. Although well intentioned, his ill-advised counsel was based on his own diagnosis, which differed from mine.

"You really should get a brain scan," Paul told me over the telephone, "because lung cancer can spread to the brain. I got one, and they found a tumor and took it out right away and I'm fine now."

"But my tumor is small, and my bone scan was clear," I said.

"You should still get one."

After my tumor was removed and doctors found no cancer cells in my lymph nodes, Paul called again. "Did you get that yet?"

"There's no reason to believe it has spread to my brain," I said, but his words were now tattooed on my thalamus. It was dreadful: I had just been hospitalized for a week after major surgery, and had spent the previous month getting scanned, probed, prodded, and tested in and around every orifice and over almost every inch of my body. I needed a break.

My friend had an answer for everything and concern that I was getting the "right" medical treatment and that I had searched for enough second opinions. I know she loved me and wanted to help, but I felt she was undermining my intelligence and treatment program. I avoided her and her "superiority of knowledge." Her actions added to my depression.

—H.D., colon cancer survivor

I emailed Paul and told him he was scaring me and not to call anymore. But it took all of my strength to communicate that, because I was so vulnerable and weak. Yet even after I asserted myself, his words haunted me.

I decided the only way to exorcise his advice was to take it. I had to wait several weeks for the MRI, during which time I suffered headaches (likely psychosomatic), imagining tumors crowding out my brain.

I was fine.

When withholding advice can heal

Margaret Stauffer's mother was not going to be fine. Stauffer joined the Wellness Community (now The Cancer Support Community) as a marriage and family therapist after reading comedienne and ovarian cancer patient Gilda Radner's book, *It's Always Something*.

When I drove to the agency's facility in Walnut Creek, California, to interview Stauffer, I expected to hear stories from her experience working with survivors, but instead, heard what I would hear from almost every authority I consulted for this book, a personal tale from her own life that helped her truly understand and better support others facing similar challenges. Stauffer shared the story of her sweet mother who endured the rigors of breast cancer three times but never talked about her fears or poor prognosis. She did share her anger, though.

"When my mother was dealing with her third recurrence of breast cancer, I remember a lot of well-meaning friends bringing her books about what she should do to recover from cancer. And I think she always had the feeling that people thought if she would just do all the things they suggested that she would be okay.

"She felt really awful about being encouraged to try so many things when she was barely hanging on to being able to do what she thought was appropriate as far as medical treatment and managing her stress and dealing with the emotions of having a third recurrence."

Stauffer said her mother had no intention of trying what her friends suggested. "She didn't want that. She had her own ideas. For her, the most important thing was being able to have music, to express herself through that—she was a pianist—and to enjoy the beauty that she saw around her."

I don't like it when anyone starts a sentence with "you have to." I loathe people telling me about alternative medicine or giving me any unsolicited medical advice.

—M.L., pituitary tumor survivor

If you want your friends or loved ones to enjoy whatever they find meaningful or beautiful in their life, give them an opportunity to tell you what they want. And if you feel the need to give advice, or fix the situation, ask permission first.

But often we don't need fixing, or if we do, we need our medical-care providers to focus on that. Dr. Rachel Naomi Remen wrote in "In the Service of Life," an article in *Noetic Sciences Review*, that if you see yourself as a fixer, you may sit in judgment, and that can preclude your truly serving. "When we fix others, we may not see their hidden wholeness or trust the integrity of life in them. Fixers trust their own expertise. When we serve, we see the unborn wholeness in others; we collaborate with it and strengthen it. Others may then be able to see their wholeness for themselves for the first time."

I know that all intentions were good but [I didn't want people] giving me advice and telling me what I should and shouldn't do without understanding my specific cancer diagnosis. Example: "You should eat lots of fruits and vegetables." I was diagnosed with colon cancer at twenty-nine and after radiation treatment, eating all that would cause nonstop diarrhea.

—D.D., colon cancer

Sometimes the suffering simply need comfort. *Merriam-Webster* defines comfort as "to give strength and hope to; to ease the grief or trouble of." How can we best do this without offering wise words that may fall flat because the pain in question is beyond words? That's when gestures become the most important form of comfort. When I think of comfort, I see a mother with babe in arms, rocking slowly, humming softly, murmuring words more as sounds, "There, there . . . it's okay."

In *The Art of Conversation Through Serious Illness*, authors Richard P. McQuellon and Michael A. Cowan discuss much more than conversation. In the chapter about personal virtues that are most needed in "mortal time," they write about gestures such as a hug or what they call "kind eyes."

"To look on another's suffering with kind eyes is to take that suffering into one's heart and hold it there gently."

⌐⌐⌐

I could not offer kind eyes to my cousin Khelly when she called me one weekday morning in 2009 soon after her forty-first birthday.

"Hey, Lor. I just found out the 'C' word isn't what I used to think," she said, referring to the vulgarity describing an anatomical part. I thought I heard a smile, but knew something dark lay beneath. "There's a word that's much worse: cancer."

My redheaded beauty of a second cousin, whose wisdom rendered her more like an elder sister even though she was my junior, had breast cancer.

This new mom and I now shared one more thing in common besides ancestors and careers in film production.

"I haven't told many people yet," she said, "but already almost everyone's giving me advice about what I should or shouldn't do, like they don't trust me! It's making me crazy! What should I do?"

I believe that most people have the answers to such questions within themselves, just as most people truly do know how to best support someone with cancer or who faces a similarly traumatic life challenge. As Dr. Marty Rossman wrote in *The Worry Solution*, "Wisdom tends to appear in the spaces between our thoughts." I agree, and encourage people struggling with such decisions to quiet themselves in meditation or prayer to access their inner wisdom. But I knew Khel needed not just answers; she needed to feel heard and understood.

She talked and I listened for almost an hour. I promised to send her a list of resources, including links to websites for young adults with cancer and email addresses of success-story survivors who I thought she could relate to. And I offered one piece of advice.

"If at all possible, I encourage you to be honest with your friends and family about what would be most helpful. They love you and need guidance—they'd want to know how much their advice is upsetting you. That said, I know how hard it can be to express that."

Five days later, I got an MP3 audio file via email that she sent to her family and friends. In her characteristically loving, but straightforward manner, she said:

"Good morning. I've got a lot on my mind, so hopefully you are open to hearing all of it. First of all, I want to thank everybody for their concern. And I'm going to have to ask you to accept and support my journey and understand that this is my journey. Let's just take a second to think about our experiences, collectively as humanity. A lot of [your] emails are concerned about me not doing conventional treatment, and I never said I wasn't going to do conventional treatment."

Khelly, who was exploring complementary, integrative, and conventional cancer treatments, went on to ask us to consider whether we had known someone who had tried chemo and survived, and whether we'd known someone who tried chemo and had not. Same for alternative treatments.

"So the question really is, 'What really works?' And you know what? Nobody knows."

She went on to share more thoughts about her cancer, and then made a request that, although still loving, belied the frustration and anger that had been building over the past week.

"I'm gonna have to ask everybody not to cram your paradigm onto mine, because it's just not helping. I find that I'm more obsessed with being angry with those emails and feeling upset and unsupported, and that's not really going to help me at all. And so, if I could ask you to do that, that would be great. And that goes the same for anyone saying to me, 'You can't do chemo and you can't do radiation,' because I can do that and that's on my list.

It hurt to hear, "You know cancer is caused by stress," "You really should do something about your relationship with X," "You should . . . you should. . . ."

—P.B., tongue cancer survivor

"So just try and be supportive and ask me how I'm feeling and tell me that I'm going to be fine, and that's really what I need from you. I hope you understand and don't take offense, but this is a really weird journey and luckily most of you haven't been on it, thankfully. I love you guys, thank you, bye."

I wasn't surprised by Khelly's reasoned and honest plea or her later request in an audio file a few days later asking us to keep our texts and emails coming, but not to expect an answer. This was a woman who was raised with a clear sense of who she was, a woman self-assured and comfortable asserting her needs. Nonetheless, she hurt as deeply as all of us do when she felt that her need for comfort was being superseded by her family's need to advise her.

Khelly was an intelligent and skilled researcher with a master's degree in communication, a positive-thinking-look-on-the-bright-side skeptic who could hold both parts of herself simultaneously. I knew that she had seen the best conventional doctors and integral care providers on the continent. I couldn't give her medical advice, which is not what she asked of me, but I did give her something to soothe her soul. With kind eyes that I hope she felt, I said, "I know you'll figure this out, Khelly."

13.

"I am still me;
treat me kindly, not differently."

I am treating you as my friend, asking you to share my present minuses
in the hope that I can ask you to share my future pluses.

—Katherine Mansfield

ALL OF US PLAY NUMEROUS ROLES IN LIFE, as parents, partners, children, colleagues, friends, and foes, often concurrently. But when most of us hear we have cancer, all other identities vanish behind the one that eclipses them: cancer patient. (We're not typically prone to call ourselves survivors yet.)

When I heard, "You have cancer," everything changed in a heartbeat. My career seemed trivial, even though just days before I beamed with pride at a recent success. Now "success" meant something entirely different: survival. I could no longer think of myself as a writer, producer, consultant, mother, or wife. *Lori Hope, CancerGal*: that was me.

Cancer changes most people profoundly and in ways that defy description. I could no longer look in the mirror and even imagine the woman I had been before. But even though I could neither see nor be the old me, I did not want to be *treated* differently. As psychologist Lawrence LeShan, said, "For

I didn't want to be treated any differently, which is why I decided to wear a wig so no one would know about my ongoing treatment unless I chose to tell them.

—R.L., breast cancer survivor

God's sake, don't wrap me in cotton batting and say, 'You poor dear thing, let me take care of you!' More people have died suffocated in cotton batting than from cancer."

Jeff Kane urges caregivers to see the whole person, not just the illness. In *How to Heal,* Dr. Kane wrote, "To the extent we see the sick person as a 'patient,' we'll relate to his patienthood instead of his wider identity. In particular, we'll undervalue his strengths. While he's sick, remember, he's unusually vulnerable to the opinions of others, so if we see him as a helpless victim, he's likely to see himself that way, too."

Dr. Kane said that evading frames that other people want to hang on cancer patients becomes more difficult when the common press jargon around cancer reporting, terms like "victim," "lost his valiant battle," and "survivor" persist. A recent Google search of "heroic battle with cancer" yielded 63,700 hits; "cancer victim" yielded more than eight million. Certainly such frames reinforce the difference between "us" and "them," and make cancer survivors special, albeit not in a good way. Such expressions simply create chasms when, more than anything, we need connection.

The kindest acts

Maria not only felt like a victim, she wondered whether she was a perpetrator and had given herself cancer. Uterine cancer is hormone-induced, and she had taken hormones. She, like many with the disease, took responsibility for something that is an act of science or nature, not of self or God.

Six days after surgery, she had enough energy to go out for a couple of hours, so asked a friend to take her to a yarn store. "I wanted to knit something for each member of my family before I died," she wrote. [This was eleven years ago, and she was still alive and doing very well!] Her friend knew it was a bit too soon for an outing but took her anyway. "There were no negative comments about feelings," said Judy. "[My friend] said, 'Okay, when do you want to go? She also helped me look for yarn . . . and acted as if we were having fun. I really couldn't decide on much and got very tired. After a bit, she helped me get back to the car. She never told me I should not be out or up or that I wasn't going to die."

Judy's friend accepted her as herself. She allowed her the freedom to see herself as a victim, but also to reach out beyond that. By showing such love, Judy's friend helped her live.

Having cancer doesn't make me a hero

Are cancer survivors valiant? Do they deserve to be placed on a pedestal for doing what any of us would do in the same situation, fight to survive? All of us emerge from the womb with a will to live; and most of us die with that will intact. We are hard-wired for it. So to revere us for simply living can seem dismissive of the real battles we're waging, and may feel condescending.

When my friend and fellow author, Kairol Rosenthal, wrote a piece in 2009 about the expression, "You're so strong!" for her blog, it caught the eye of *New York Times* journalist Tara Parker-Pope, who consequently asked her readers, "Does cancer make you strong?" The response from 159 readers was, in nearly every case, a resounding "No!" But one person, in fact the first to comment, asked sarcastically, "So, should people say, 'Gosh, you have reacted in an utterly uninspiring and routine way to tragic circumstances about which you had no control?' Surely, there are some cancer patients who exhibit strength and grace and deserve to be credited for it."

Parker-Pope answered, "Of course not. But it's also not the responsibility of people with cancer to inspire us or set an example. I think the point is that by focusing on strength and grace, we may deny people the opportunity to be weak, to crumble and to cry and to curse their disease."

> *My husband was awesome. The thing I really was thankful for was the fact that he allowed me to do "normal" things, like wash dishes, of all things. He didn't fuss over me when I attempted to do things I probably shouldn't have done, he just allowed me to do things as normally as possible.*
>
> —T.A., breast cancer survivor

Beyond the crumble and the curse

Even before John could read, his two most prized possessions were books: one was about taking a trip on a passenger plane, the other, a children's encyclopedia that included illustrations of a pilot flying an airplane: "Push the wheel, houses get bigger. Pull the wheel, houses get smaller," John's mother read to him. "Those words and seeing the movie *Airport* on TV fueled a vivid fantasy of me being "The Kid Who Saved that Jetliner by Taking the Controls When the Pilots Ate the Bad Fish."

But what really propelled John to learn how to fly was a summer class about airplanes he took at a local museum when he was twelve. "It concluded with a flight up front in a real airplane, a Beechcraft V35 Bonanza, and I got to try my hand at the controls. Sure enough, I pushed the yoke and the houses got bigger. Pulled the yoke back and the houses got smaller. I was hooked!"

Never one to shrink from a challenge, John learned to pilot at a tiny 2000-foot strip with trees in the approach path. Though he worked full-time, he always made time to fly, earning his private pilot's certificate in nine months.

People don't change when they get cancer and suddenly stop wanting to be called smart, sexy, fun, funny, a good Christian, an excellent cook, singer, etc. or a total fashionista. People are more than their cancer.

—F.T., thyroid cancer survivor

He loved flying not just for the fun, but for the freedom it afforded. I understood, because I became a pilot in my twenties, and it both lifted my confidence and gave me the freedom to return to earth after a wild ride of indecision about my career. John loved all aspects of the freedom. "Being able to move around in all three dimensions, unobstructed, and above a carpet of beautiful scenery is always liberating. Liberating mentally, too. Because flying safely takes 100 percent of your concentration and attention, all your outside worries disappear."

But while his spirits soared, his body had been secretly spiraling downward. His lymph nodes had swelled to the size of peach pits. Less than one month after receiving his license, he received a diagnosis of Hodgkin's lymphoma.

"Okay, now the real adventure begins," he remembered thinking. He had every possible medical test to determine the stage of his illness, which would determine his treatment, and surgeons removed the enlarged lymph node in his neck. He was awake during the procedure, because he says his insurance would not pay for general anesthesia. He heard the surgeon say to him, as he removed the largest node. "You just won the Olympics of lymph nodes." Always the joker, John asked, "You mean the *Olymphics*?"

John underwent grueling chemotherapy and radiation, but he continued to pilot throughout his treatment.

"I used to fly (always with an instructor aboard), and from the minute I took off until a good three hours after I landed, it was the only time I was totally pain-free."

The most painful part of his cancer experience was the way people behaved around him. Although his boss did not treat him differently and never called attention to his illness, his family did.

"I needed to do certain things for myself. I wanted to cook for myself, and I wanted to play tennis. My dad came to visit and was trying to cook for me and everything. Finally I had to tell him to go home."

John said his father's solicitude made him feel different from and "less than" his peers. Once he was free of his father and others who coddled him and treated him like a patient, he felt normal again and resumed his old life, which included flying solo.

"Surviving cancer just reinforced the great feelings I already had about flying. I think flying actually changed my feelings about cancer more than vice versa. Learning to fly is an often daunting and discouraging task that requires lots of effort and study and transforming self-doubt into self-confidence. It's all driven by hope, survival instinct, personal drive, encouragement from others and perseverance toward a goal. When it came to fighting cancer, I'd already been through the drill."

> *Treat us like we are still normal. We may be sick, or we may have been ill, but we are still the same people we were before cancer. Don't look at us with pity in your eyes or voice. Don't be patronizing.*
>
> —D.F., prostate cancer survivor

Monica, whom you met in chapter 12, wanted to fly, too—as a passenger. Shortly after completing treatment, she wanted to attend a professional conference she had been looking forward to for months, but several friends cautioned her not to go because she would have to fly on an airplane and expose herself to germs.

"Sometimes you just want to forget and not be the patient," she said. "One of the reasons I wanted to go to the conference is so I could just be a person. I went there and no one said, 'It's 1 a.m., shouldn't you be going to bed now?' I got to be a regular person."

People often give me credit for being a long-term survivor. I wish I could explain that it truly has little to do with me personally, but it's the make up of my cancer. It is relatively slow growing and responds well to treatments. I think people would rather believe that I possess some ability to control the progression of the cancer and give me credit for something I have little to do with. It makes me uncomfortable.

—S.P., lung cancer survivor

But even once you are "cured," many people still think of you as a cancer survivor. When my cousin Barbara reached her five-year survival date, she no longer chose to call herself a cancer survivor. "I've had many things happen in my past that I don't identify myself in terms of because they're no longer part of me," she wrote, "and cancer is one such thing. For example, I was divorced, but don't consider myself a divorcée. I had measles, but I don't consider myself a measles survivor. I used to be a waitress, but I don't consider myself an ex-waitress."

But shaking the label of waitress is easier than losing "cancer survivor." A stigma often persists, affording the disease more power than it deserves, especially when one is still battling it.

"They have a disease, but they're still the same person, and to change the way you react to or interact with that person makes the disease more important than what attracted you to that person in the first place," observed Bay Area Tumor Institute director, Barry Siegel.

What's crucial is to remember that people with cancer are people first, and that by focusing on who they are as individuals and what they might need, specifically, you can best help them live.

14.

"If you really want to help me, be specific about your offer, or just help without asking."

Say yes when nobody asked.

—Lao proverb

IN THE ACADEMY AWARD–NOMINATED FILM *Winter's Bone*, hungry and near-homeless teenager Ree and her twelve-year-old brother Sonny are watching their neighbors cut up a deer carcass. The brother says, "Maybe they'll share some of that with us."

"That could be," answers Ree.

"Maybe we should ask."

Ree holds his face in her hands, looks straight into his eyes, and says slowly, "Never ask for what oughta be offered."

↩↩↩

One afternoon after undergoing a PET scan in the morning to see if there were signs of cancer beyond my lungs, I went to get my bangs trimmed. When I plopped in the leather-look chair, I divulged what I'd been through that morning, sharing with the stylist that I had cancer and would soon undergo major surgery. She said something about how awful it was, and shook her head slowly, with a "tsk, tsk."

My friend said, "If you need anything—someone to clean toilets or punch around to blow off some stress—I'm available this coming Tuesday." It made me feel like laughing, because it was an offer, but I didn't have to make a real commitment. She was there if I need her, but she wouldn't be hurt if I didn't.

—S.M., uterine cancer survivor

I watched protectively as she ran the special thinning scissors through my bangs, fearing she would cut too much. My worry enlarged through the lens of imminent test results. When my cell phone rang a few minutes later, my hand bolted to the counter.

"Lori, there are several areas of your PET scan that show increased metabolic activity," said my surgeon.

I saw the reflection of my face turning white, as blood rushed to my racing heart.

"Where?" I demanded.

"In your abdominal area."

The heat of tears. "What does that mean? Has the cancer spread?"

"You need to come in so we can talk about this," he said curtly.

"But I need to know!"

"This is not something we can talk about now," he insisted.

"But. . . ." *Deep breaths*, I told myself. "Okay," I surrendered, too weak to challenge the man who would soon literally hold my life in his hands and hopefully save it.

"Can you come in tomorrow morning at ten?" he asked.

When I hung up, I wanted to scream, but instead asked what I owed the stylist for the thinning she had yet to finish.

"Five dollars."

Trembling, I rummaged through my purse for my wallet, while the stylist waited, silent. I finally pulled out a crisp five, left it on the counter, and dashed out in tears.

I loved it when friends would call each other about what I needed instead of me having to make the phone call when I felt so terrible. Wow, I had incredible friends!

—S.R., skin cancer survivor

On my way home, my mind was a washing machine spinning through cycles of terror and anger. I desperately needed nurturing, kindness, and comfort. If only the stylist had said, "Don't worry about paying" or even "I'm so sorry—it sounds like you got some bad news." Instead, the words, "Five dollars" burned in my mind like acid.

She meant no harm, and I suspect she had no idea how I felt or what I needed. Perhaps she was shocked and scared herself, or perhaps she was desperate for money. But, still, she missed an opportunity to make a mammoth difference with the most simple gesture of kindness.

Instead of asking can I do anything, just do something, don't wait for me or my caregiver to ask, because we more than likely won't.

—G.H., renal cell cancer survivor

Gestures: make them simple, not empty

One male respondent to my survey offered this comment: "No empty gestures. If you offer to do something, follow through with it. That simple. Whether you're offering to drive me to a doctor appointment or do my yard work or let me sleep with your wife, just make sure you follow through."

Why is this so important? For many, requesting and accepting help can be difficult enough, but once they do open themselves up, people with cancer can be doubly disappointed when others let them down. They already feel like they're standing on cliff edge that could give at any moment and may berate themselves for asking in the first place. It may make it more dangerous to trust that friend, and perhaps others, down the line.

I'm one of those people who find it challenging to ask for help. I trace it back to my teens. When my father left my mother, I, too, felt abandoned. Perhaps because I was older and appeared to be so independent, no one (at least no one in memory) was there to support me. Nor was my mother, who tried to commit suicide at the kitchen table while I struggled to take away the pastel pills she'd spilled out in front of her like little breath mints. I called her psychiatrist and he persuaded her to let me drive her to the hospital.

I learned to be self-sufficient. And to put up a good, strong front.

"You're so amazing," my father's new, mostly younger friends would marvel, as I charmed them with wise words. But inside I felt neither sagacious nor strong. Simply alone. And for years a part of me expected to be left alone, and I likely pushed people away because of it. Ultimately I did learn to trust, partly because by my late thirties I had matured and met a man, my husband and best friend, David, who was present for me in body, mind, spirit, heart, and soul like no one else had ever been.

When I had cancer, almost everyone I cared about showed up for me. But one neighbor who stopped by for a visit and offered enthusiastically, "I'm here to help in any way I can, just call me, anytime!" denied my request when I finally marshaled the emotional strength to push the seven digits on my phone. It was a few weeks after my surgery, and I still lacked the stamina I thought would return long before.

I liked it when friends said, "Here is my email address; add me to your Meals on Wheels list, or your child care list or your clean your house list." Some friends simply took the initiative to start these lists themselves and that was fine, too.

—M.J., acute myeloid leukemia survivor

"Hi, Dienie," I recorded with false cheer on her cell phone voicemail. "You offered to help me a while back and I could really use it today. I'm exhausted and just can't make it to the store. Can you give me a call please?"

"Gosh, Lori, sorry, I can't help you today," she apologized when she finally called back, hours later. "I have to pick up my son at school and then take him to practice. Hope you can find someone else."

"It was hard enough to pick up the phone once and ask for help, and I don't have the energy to call someone else," I could have said, adding, "And if you weren't willing to go out of your way to help, why did you offer?" But instead, I reassured her not to feel bad, then crawled back into bed, buried my head in the pillows, let the sobs shake me, then ordered take-out.

"How can I help?"

If you haven't had cancer or suffered from a disabling or chronic disease, or had a newborn, or had a close family member die, you may reflexively ask a friend or loved one in such a situation, "How can I help?" Or, not knowing how to help, you might offer, "Call me if you need anything."

But even making a specific offer can backfire if you're not willing to make good on it. And making a nondescript offer or asking with all good intentions how you can help without taking time to imagine what could really make a difference, can add to the burden of someone already shouldering a huge load. When you have cancer, everything else fades in the background. Your mind, muddled by emotions and hormones, may skew your sense of what matters, and preclude knowing what you need in order to function.

Food? "Not hungry."

Exercise? "I'm running from cancer as fast I can."

Clean clothes? "Oh, those. . . ."

Asking someone who may feel overwhelmed with often literal life-and-death decisions about what they need is not what they need. It's kinder to ask specifically, "Can I pick up your son from soccer practice? Can I take him out to eat so you can have some time with your husband?" Or "Can I pick up your laundry and do it for you?" Or "I'm going to the grocery store: can I pick up some food for you?" (See more specific suggestions in part II.)

Sometimes you have to be more proactive and ask more than once. Psychologist Paul Ekman says it's crucial to consider your audience when deciding how assertive to be.

"I have one friend who is quite a close friend, but he's such a reserved person that I can never expect him to call me when he's ill, even though he's not married and he has no children," Dr. Ekman said. "I'm one of the few people, when he gets a treatment and someone has to take him home, whom he can ask. There aren't many people like that, but I have to tell him again and again, 'I want to!' because he won't take more initiative."

> *Someone with cancer is too overwhelmed, tired, or sick to reach out and call people to ask for help. Friends should call the patient, and ask when the next doctor's appointment is, and offer to drive the patient, or sit with them during chemo.*
>
> —J.D., breast cancer

乙乙乙

Although most people appreciate receiving help without having to strain their imagination, arranging for un-asked-for support can backfire. My neighbor Nancy emailed me about an example of an unusual "blunder," as she called it.

"My colleague, a former reporter named Mary, was writing speeches when she was diagnosed with stage 3 breast cancer at age forty-four. She and her husband had gone to Peru four years earlier to adopt a Peruvian infant when he was just a few weeks old." The baby fulfilled the couple's longtime dream.

When Mary learned she had cancer, she was shattered, fearing she would leave her son motherless. She underwent a bone marrow transplant, and Nancy and her colleagues wanted to help by organizing shifts of people to clean her house, help with child care, shop, and cook. Nancy was designated to offer their services but was completely unprepared for Mary's response. "She wanted nothing from us; she was insulted and furious. 'I can pay someone to clean my house,' she said. 'I know you want to help, but I can't take care of your needs."

Nancy felt horrible. "To have approached Mary full of love and to have made her feel worse was devastating. Over time I have come to understand her response, I think; one of the things [people like Mary] must cope with is being totally out of control. Rejecting our offer and arranging for her own help might have given her back some control and dignity. Maybe sometimes there is no comfort that can come from the outside."

> A friend's teenaged daughters planted flowers in my garden without my asking. They were beautiful!
>
> —T.J., ovarian cancer survivor

That may be true, sometimes, but that story spoke to me of the importance of asking permission. If there is any shred of doubt, it is best to ask. That goes for helping a blind person across the street, opening a door for someone in a wheelchair, or bringing a pot of soup to a family with cancer.

The only thing you do not need to ask permission for is to silently send good thoughts or love.

15.
"I love being held in your thoughts or prayers."

Prayer doesn't change things; it changes people, and they change things.

—Anonymous

SIXTY-THREE-YEAR-OLD ARTIE GOLDEN suspected a bladder infection when he needed to urinate frequently and experienced a burning sensation while doing so. Instead, it was bladder cancer. He had no tumors and therefore didn't warrant surgery but instead underwent an unusual treatment. Although it was more than six years ago, Artie recounted almost every detail.

"I got this live tuberculin bacillus injected into my bladder each week," he began. "The bladder detects a substance and tries to slough off cells. They put fifty cc's into the bladder, and then have you lay on your left side fifteen minutes, then your right side, then your back and front, swishing it around."

Pepto-Bismol commercials came to mind. I was fascinated that such a high tech treatment could rely on something as fundamental as gravity.

Artie continued, "You go home and hold it for one hour, and then urinate." I remembered getting a pelvic ultrasound exam after my positive PET scan and enduring the torture of a full bladder while the tech rolled the rounded metal nub over my tummy looking for other tumors.

Many, many friends said they kept me in their prayers—that felt wonderful!

—N.N., breast cancer survivor

"Then you treat the toilet with Clorox. There's a cure rate of 80 percent . . . and I had great results," he sighed. "Except in one spot." He needed an eight-and-a-half hour operation to remove the remaining cancer.

"It was 100 percent successful. They make a bladder out of your bowel, take it out, and filet it so they can reconnect it. But my surgeon couldn't reconnect it, so I have to use a catheter every four to six hours to urinate.

"You have to live with that. Attitude is a big part of it. Let's go forward with life."

Another thing that helped him move forward was the tremendous out-pouring of love and support he received from his family and religious congregation. Though not "overly religious," he said, he believes prayer helped him heal.

"There must be some power greater than what I can discern. I went to a bar mitzvah a few months ago and I ran into a casual friend who's also a cancer survivor. He said to me, 'I come to the temple every morning and I pray for you every day.'" Artie paused. "Even now—still—six years later, he's praying for me every day! It makes you feel so great. And I really believe that has helped me survive."

The power of believing in someone

Soon after Carol was diagnosed with cancer, she emailed almost everyone she knew, requesting that they send good thoughts or prayers. She knew she needed all the support she could get, and felt no shame in asking for it. Carol received hundreds of emails, calls, and greeting cards from friends, acquaintances, colleagues, and friends of friends and even a few strangers. Everyone encouraged, assured, or buoyed her hopes, except for one person.

"An old friend from grade school, Brandon, emailed me and said he wasn't going to pray for me, because he didn't believe prayer was effective. He was a microbiologist," Carol added, "and he did say he would send all love my way."

He also sent a bouquet of white lilies. "Their sweet, strong fragrance stuck in my nasal hairs—just like his refusal to pray for me stuck in my heart," Carol said.

"As much as I appreciated his love and respected his right to his opinion, Brandon's comment pierced me." She wanted to believe the prayers would make a difference, and even though she believed thoughts, love, and prayer similar in purpose, she did believe there was something different about prayer. She had attended the Harvard University School of Continuing Education's Spirituality and Healing in Medicine conference with Herbert Benson, MD, a pioneer in mind-body medicine and the creator of the Relaxation Response. And she kept up with the latest on healing. A recent study showed that patients in a coronary care unit who were prayed for had significantly fewer complications. But another study—the one Carol's grammar school friend cited—had shown prayer had no influence.

"I understood that. With his background, of course Brandon would say that. But that's not what I needed to hear. At that point, I needed all the ammunition I could gather, every force I could bring to bear, not just to fight my cancer, but to keep my head and heart above water."

I had one teacher just tell me she didn't need to know what was happening, but she was praying for me. That meant a lot, because I knew she wasn't going to gossip about it and was coming from a sincere place.

—T.T., thyroid cancer survivor

Like many people who feel particularly vulnerable, Carol also fell victim to superstition. Gandhi said, "Prayers are no superstitions; they are more real than the acts of eating, drinking, sitting, or walking." But to Carol, superstition and prayer went hand in hand. "Even though I don't believe in a thumbs-up/thumbs-down God with a gray beard who makes decisions on a case-by-case basis, I thought of my cancer as an election of sorts. The more votes—meaning the more prayers—the better."

Carol called Brandon to thank him for the beautiful flowers and love he sent, and brought up the subject of prayer. "I thought I was just curious; I respected his opinion, and we had always had interesting conversations.

"But," she continued, "I suspect I may have just wanted to be right. I wanted Brandon to agree with me. Instead, he dug in his heels. 'I'm sorry. I just don't believe that prayer can heal people,' he insisted. 'I've read the studies, and they're just not conclusive.'

"What I realized after our conversation was that I not only wanted to believe that prayer works, but I also wanted him to care enough about me to stretch a little, reach out, maybe even misrepresent his beliefs."

Perhaps Brandon could have said, "A lot of studies do support that notion."

"Would it have been so hard for him to say that?" Carol asked. "Part of me still feels angry. But the other part knows he loves me. He not only said so, he showed it, over and over, with flowers, greeting cards, and other symbols."

Fact is, when you feel that weak and vulnerable, you do not want conflict. Although Carol did invite confrontation, she wanted Brandon's support. "He undermined my faith, and although I know that was not at all his intention, that was the effect."

> *I also wanted people to pray for me—I asked everyone to keep me in their prayers and I feel like it made a huge difference in my outcome!*
>
> —J.M., soft tissue sarcoma survivor

What is prayer?

In the Help Me Live Cancer Support Survey, the statement, "I love being kept in your thoughts or prayers" was rated third, just behind "I am more grateful than I can say for your care, compassion, and support," and "I need to laugh—or just forget about cancer for a while."

Clearly, people need and want to know that they matter and that others are doing something, if only thinking about them, to prove it. So perhaps Carol was asking the wrong question. Perhaps instead of asking whether prayer worked, she should have asked herself what prayer is and what function it serves.

In his book *When Bad Things Happen to Good People*, Rabbi Harold Kushner asked what we are doing when we pray to God for a favorable outcome. Do we really believe in a God who has the power to cure malignancies and influence the outcome of surgery? "And if we don't get what we prayed for, how do we keep from being either angry with God or feeling that we have been judged and found wanting?"

Rabbi Kushner explained what he prays for when someone is ill, giving an example of a time when a stranger called him and asked him to pray for his mother who was about to undergo surgery. "Why did I agree, if I don't believe that my prayers (or his for that matter) will move God to affect the results . . . ? By agreeing, I was saying to him, 'I understand that you are worried and afraid of what might happen. I want you to know that I, and your neighbors in this community, share that concern. We are with you, even though we don't know you, because we can imagine ourselves being in your situation and wanting and needing all the support we can get. We are hoping and praying along with you that things turn out well, so that you don't have to feel that you are facing this frightening situation alone. . . .'

"Prayer, when it is offered in the right way, redeems people from isolation."

"I don't think it's possible to overrate sick people's need for attention," wrote physician Jeff Kane in *How to Heal.* He said people in his cancer support group have been telling him that for years. "When we feel recognized, witnessed, and understood, we shine. We feel tangibly better: recognition is a major healing stimulant, on a par, I'd say, with adequate sleep. If closeness promotes healing," he continued, "then we're asking for trouble when we increase distance."

> *I have a tremendous faith in God and I really had to keep reminding myself to give it up to the Higher Power. My friends and family know this and helped me to stay connected to my beliefs.*
>
> —R.Y., kidney cancer survivor

When Brandon argued with Carol, she felt he put distance between them. "I needed him to stay close, even though he was thousands of miles away."

When I had cancer, my cousin Barbara contacted a group of religious women at a convent who agreed to pray for me night and day. My congregation at Alameda's Temple Israel said a *mi sheberach* (a traditional healing prayer) every week for me at Friday night services, while my Christian friends offered their own prayers. My nonreligious friends and my medical doctor, a Buddhist, meditated on my healing. My friend Nasus performed a Native American sage smudge on my home to purify it and promote healing. Although I did not know a sage smudge from sandalwood incense, I felt the love as surely as I smelled the musky smoke that permeated my furniture. The love was tangible, and it brought much comfort.

But prayer doesn't always assuage anxiety, as Mary explained when she told the story of her son Peter and his wife.

"My daughter-in-law is dying of cancer," she said, her voice quieting almost to a whisper. "What she and my son have been going through is so hard. People will look at them and say, 'Well, I'm praying for you.' There's a kind of sense that you're already dead.

"There's an implication here that's very hard to tolerate," Mary continued. "My son told me, 'I thank people, I appreciate their prayers, but I'd probably just rather people say, 'I'm hanging in there for you' or 'I'm thinking about you.'"

"I'm praying for you" might mean something altogether different to Mary and Peter once their beloved has died. "And that's one of the problems," said Brother Daniel, a monk whose work is to pray at New Camaldoli silent monastery and retreat center. "For people who don't pray much, it can be frightening when they hear that other people are praying for them. Some people associate praying only with funerals. And that's why it scares them."

I told my surgeon that I believe in the power of prayer, and told her I was praying for her and her team and I wanted her to pray, too, if she was comfortable doing so. She said, "I believe in the power of prayer," and squeezed my hand. I went into surgery calmly and optimistically.

—M.E., colon cancer survivor

Whether prayer improves health or not, whether it's desired or not, virtually everyone appreciates feeling as if they matter and are loved. It's wise to consider your audience, and your friend or loved one's spiritual beliefs, and it may be best to ask permission—"May I pray for you? Would you like that?"—before telling someone you're sending mental telegrams to the Great Upstairs. But if you have love to send, you don't need to ask. Just feel it. And let your friend or loved one know it. More than any other statement in my survey of more than six hundred cancer survivors, "I love you" was the one most people said they yearn to hear.

16.

"Hearing platitudes or what's good about cancer can minimize my feelings."

Sooner throw a pearl at hazard than an idle or useless word.

—Pythagoras

"HE'S IN A BETTER PLACE NOW," said a funeral attendee to Trish, referring to her husband. "A better place would be in my arms," Trish wanted to rejoin.

"Some people say, 'You can use cancer to transform your life,' said Jane, a cancer survivor. "Well, as they say in psychotherapy, A-F-O-G— 'another f-ing opportunity for growth!'" she chuckled. "I transformed my life a long time ago—I already went through a horrible divorce. It's not like I needed a kick in the butt. People saying that just ticks me off."

Platitudes are often voiced without thought; they come to mind easily because they're "tried and true"—except of course, when they're not. "God doesn't give you more than you can handle"—but what about people who commit suicide?

Though well intentioned, such clichés may come across as insincere or dismissive,

> It's hard to explain that it does feel different from your normal, statistical risk of being hit by a car.
>
> —A.B., breast cancer survivor

133

making light of life's most onerous experiences. To a soul rendered raw by trauma and in need of comfort and compassion, platitudes sting partly because they sound generic and don't take into consideration the individual's unique situation. Platitudes add distance and often betray a lack of compassion. It's safer and easier to throw bromides between you and another instead of truly listening and risking the penetration of pain—even though providing such compassion often results in genuine and lasting satisfaction.

People always say to me, well, any of us could get hit by a car today and die, so I interpret that as, "What's the big deal?" The reality is that I am in a higher risk category.

—D.A., lung cancer survivor

As psychologist Paul Ekman said, people in pain need someone capable of emotional empathy to reverberate what they're feeling. But some people simply cannot relate, and that's partly why they proffer platitudes. As noted earlier, Dr. Ekman said some people, have a restrictive range of emotions and cannot deal with bad news or sick people. They might do well to send greeting cards in lieu of unwelcome words. (Though some greeting cards are rife with trite and not necessarily helpful sayings.)

Although a cliché to one person may be a truth to another, some common sayings seem to strike many cancer survivors as inappropriate, as confirmed by my survey of more than six hundred cancer survivors. In the following pages, I outline some of those sayings in the hope that you will think twice before speaking them. They may not be offensive to your loved one—again, survivors often differ—and if you feel compelled to offer the words anyway, you might preface them with "I hope this doesn't trivialize what you're going through, but I'd like to offer a saying that means a lot to me."

"Any of us could get hit by a bus!"

The platitude many cancer survivors report disliking most is "I could go outside and get hit by a bus/truck/car/train/meteor!" Many have heard at least one version of this. "I heard that maybe ten times, even by my primary care physician," said Johanna, whose lymphoma threatened her life of twenty-seven years. "It was kind of like, 'Okay, so then in addition to the fact that I could die from cancer, I might also get hit by a truck'!" This also implies that the patient is facing imminent death, which may be wrong and deeply disturbing to someone in need of hope.

Some patients actually say they would prefer getting flattened by a truck because that death would likely be sudden and painless. Also, being struck by cancer differs from accidentally walking into the path of a fast-moving vehicle because you can identify the moment a bus runs you over, while you can never know when exactly when cancer cells started multiplying invisibly in your body.

Although a person who says, "I could get hit by a bus" may be attempting to put herself on the same level, there's a strange irony here. Fact is, we will all die, but the difference is that people with cancer may have a better idea of when, and may be therefore better equipped to prepare and cope for the end. In any event, saying "I could get hit by a bus" may minimize the process of what happens along the way.

At least . . ."

If I had a choice, I would probably choose cancer over getting hit by a bus, and I'm not alone. National Public Radio aired a story about an oncology social worker who surveyed sixty of her peers, asking them how they would want to die. She found that almost all the respondents said they would rather die of cancer than a heart attack or in an auto crash. Few feared physical suffering, because the medical practice of palliative care has become widespread not only in oncology but throughout all medical specialties. Much more troubling was the thought of leaving things left unsaid. While terminally ill people have the opportunity to tie up loose ends and prepare to die, those who die suddenly can leave behind a bitter legacy of longing or regret.

Former First Lady Jackie Kennedy Onassis wrote to her priest, Rev. Richard McSorley, referring to her first husband's assassination, "If I only had a minute to say good-bye. . . . It was so hard not to say good-bye, not be able to say good-bye."

Yet even when you get to say good-bye, you don't want others saying, "At least you got to say good-bye," because it trivializes a deep and profound loss. Beginning a sentence with "At least. . . ," at best minimizes and at worst totally dismisses a concern or worry. A cousin of "You just have to think positively," the phrase points to the bright side, reminding you that someone else has it worse. And that you're in some way lucky. Although I wholly believe in the practice and science of gratitude and even positive psychology in most situations, I believe in compassion in all situations. "At least . . ." precludes, if only for a moment, compassion.

Also, countering your friend or loved one's suffering with "At least . . ." can also rob him of the joy of discovering the bright side himself. As discussed in chapter 8, when you allow someone to voice the negative, it often frees him to see and even celebrate the positive aspects of him situation.

My neighbor said it would take me less time to get ready since I didn't have to wash my hair. That's not what I needed to hear.

—N.W., thyroid cancer survivor

Finally, saying "At least . . ." can make you sound kind of ridiculous. One cancer survivor who answered the Help Me Live Cancer Support Survey reported that a coworker's father, who was in rehab for alcoholism, said, "[At least cancer] isn't as bad as other diseases such as alcoholism, which affects the entire family more than just the person dealing with the disease."

"Everything happens for a reason"

Patti's pet peeve is being told "This happened for a reason" or "because you can handle it." People said such things both while her husband, Louis, was suffering from multiple tumors and after he died.

"It's sort of like a pseudo-Eastern approach, which is like there's a balance in the universe and this happened for a reason," she said, still angry years later.

"I was looking at [Rabbi Harold] Kushner's book, *When Bad Things Happen to Good People*," she continued. "The book says there is chaos in the world and things just happen. So, stop!" she snapped, making a plea to those who want to tell her Louis died for a reason.

"Everything's going to be okay" or "You'll be just fine"

"You'll be fine. . . . I have a friend who had the same thing and she's fine now." That's what Janice heard from a loved one. "Nobody, including the oncologist," Janice complained, "knows if a patient will be fine. I know the statement is meant to encourage, but it trivializes the seriousness of the disease."

As psychologist Lawrence LeShan said, "Don't tell me things you don't know anything about. Don't tell me I'm going to get better, don't tell me I'm going to get worse."

Another woman, Geena, just diagnosed with breast cancer, tells the story of her friend Douglas. "Mickey Mouse is his idol. He has this little Mickey Mouse tattoo."

When she sent Douglas an email, just days after her diagnosis, he replied, electronically: "Hi, Geena. You'll be fine."

"He added a little 'blah-blah-blah,' you know, and then, 'Have a good day,'" said Geena. "And I thought, 'After what I told you, how can you imagine that I'm going to have a good day for a few more days?' Now I can laugh about it, but at that point . . ."

What hurt most about Douglas's naïve response is that it did not feel loving. "Douglas always says, 'I know what you're going through.' Or 'I know how you feel.' He always gives advice. And usually he knows nothing about what I am going through—although he can be a very good listener.

"It's isolating in a way, because it says to me he really doesn't grasp what I'm going through. It doesn't make me feel closer to him. I have to back up and remember that he loves me."

Dolores Moorehead of the Cancer Support Community says many people just don't know how to deal with the reality of their own mortality. "A lot of times I feel that when people say, 'You're going to be okay,' it's partly because that's what they need to hear—not so much what you need to hear. It makes them feel better, because they really don't know what to do with what's happening and how they're feeling."

"Cancer is a gift."

When someone suggests to Barbara Brenner that cancer is a gift, she answers, "A gift is something you would give away. To whom would you give this gift?"

And, I would add, *"What's the return policy?"*

It's bad enough to hear these words from a cancer survivor who may have discovered lessons or gifts from their disease, but when they come from someone who cannot truly know what it's like to go through this, the words can feel insulting.

When someone says, "It's God's will," I feel like it's a hopeless situation. And why would God want me to suffer like this?

—I.N., pancreatic cancer survivor

Cancer inspires soul searching and often more questions that you can never imagine. Before you ask what seems to some a logical question, "Why did you get cancer?," please read on.

17.

"I don't know why I got cancer, and hearing your theory may add grave insult to injury."

A man thinks that by mouthing hard words he understands hard things.

—Herman Melville

I SMOKED MY FIRST CIGARETTE just before the US Surgeon General declared smoking "hazardous to your health." But even knowing the true dangers may not have precluded my inhaling the noxious chemicals. I was a teen who yearned to fit in with the in-crowd and look older. I never gave much thought to actually *growing* older than my midtwenties, when, I imagined, I'd be married to my boyfriend Lanny—who taught me to smoke while we picnicked in Shaw Park on sultry St. Louis summer days—surrounded by a gaggle of kids.

I quit in the mid-1980s, long after cigarettes were upgraded from "hazardous" to "dangerous," and after numerous attempts. I was in my late twenties and not only came to detest the tobacco industry but also realized that when, as a medical reporter, I sneaked down the back stairs to the basement bathroom and

A few people act as if you might be contagious or had done something to deserve the disease. Now that really hurt, I suppose because of the little nagging voice inside that's saying the same thing.

—D.A., Hodgkin's lymphoma survivor

donned a shower cap and raincoat so I could sneak a cigarette without smelling like one, I was a true addict.

In spite of doing the "right thing" by quitting, I was diagnosed with lung cancer almost twenty years later.

"Did you smoke?" I heard again and again. The question made me feel judged, defensive, and guilty. I harbored many secret theories, as do many survivors, about why I got cancer, and most had nothing to do with cigarettes. They involved transgressions dating back to my second boyfriend, whose heart I broke. Then there was the workaholism I was so often accused of. "I must have gotten cancer because I somehow deserved it," I thought, in my superstitious, regressive state.

But it's not just regression that makes us blame ourselves. As Susan Sontag noted in her brilliant 1978 essay and analysis, "Illness as Metaphor," the pervasive and historical perception of disease as punishment, and the association of cancer with evil and the attendant metaphors used to describe diseases such as cancer, reinforce our sense of personal culpability. Sontag wrote, "Such preposterous and dangerous views manage to put the onus of the disease on the patient and not only weaken the patient's ability to understand the range of plausible medical treatment but also, implicitly, direct the patient away from such treatment."

Two different massage therapists suggested that I had brought on my own cancer through negative thoughts!! Even though I didn't believe it for a second, it outraged me that someone else believed it. Plus, it ruined the massages.

—F.P. sarcoma survivor

I believe now that I got cancer partly because I smoked, though plenty of people who smoke longer and more than I did never get lung cancer. More important, many people who never smoked get lung cancer. Like psychiatrist Jimmie Holland's daughter-in-law, who is among the 15 to 20 percent of never-smokers diagnosed with the disease. When I interviewed Dr. Holland, she told me her son's wife was dying of lung cancer. Just thirty-seven years old, she had run out of treatment options.

I asked Dr. Holland if people asked her daughter-in-law whether she smoked. "You know, I don't know," she replied. "But I find myself saying that she never smoked, which is kind of interesting; why I have to say that is interesting.

"Why did she get it?" asked Dr. Holland. "Was it in her family? No, it's not in her family. People want to establish a cause, particularly when it's a young person and it's unexpected. If you can attribute a cause then you can say, 'It won't happen to me, I don't smoke so I'm safe'—it's a sort of 'you and not me' situation. If we can figure out why it happened, well, then it won't happen to me."

When a rare form of cancer, cancer of the tonsils, happened to Jamie, he didn't blame himself. He hadn't had a drink for twenty years or smoked much, he told me, and because the disease is so rare, his friends didn't say very much about it. That was a good thing, he said, because he did not feel comfortable talking about it with anyone but his girlfriend, a singer. But that turned out not to be such a good thing.

"She said that because I didn't use my voice, my voice was being taken away from me," said Jamie. "I never had a great voice, but now I was taken a notch down. She meant this in an expressive way, not just literally, like 'You need to speak up for yourself.'

> *The most common thing was on the order of "This is something you manifested and if you figure out what the lesson is, you will be cured." Bull s**t stuff like that.*
>
> —S.T., testicular cancer survivor

"I think because she was a singer, saying that was her protection, like 'This is why it won't happen to me.' I was sitting next to her, and I just said, 'Oh.' But by the end of her saying that, she knew she was on thin ice."

Why me? Why *not* me?

Why do bad things happen to good people and good things happen to bad people? Is it God's will? Are those who smoke immoral or weak? What about obese overeaters or workaholics who give more to their jobs than their families?

"I was brought up in the Catholic faith," said Joanne, a lung cancer survivor who used to work for an AIDS food bank, "and to say that God would put down someone because of a lifestyle is just ridiculous." Joanne said that since she worked at the food bank, many people assumed she had

AIDS and looked down at her. "The rudeness of people—how could you blame someone for having it? You see the very positive and very negative side of people."

"What caused it?" upsets not only people with cancers that may have known or suspected causes. As a fifty-four-year-old survivor commented in the Help Me Live Survey, "No one wants to hear there's no known cause for sarcoma, so there's no way they can avoid a similar fate; also, there's always the undercurrent that if I'd taken better care of myself, I wouldn't be in this fix."

Beyond "why?"

I do not know how long I had cancer before it was diagnosed. I showed no symptoms: the very small tumor was discovered by mistake—or Providence—when I got a CT scan of my abdomen for an unrelated condition. I certainly started growing the tumor after I quit smoking—a recent study by the University of North Carolina School of Medicine estimates that most solid lung, breast, and colon cancer tumors have existed for three to six years before they are detected—but perhaps the genetic damage was done during my years as a smoker. What made my tumor grow? Guilt? Polluted air? Radon, the second biggest cause of lung cancer, causing 21,000 lung cancer deaths yearly in this country?

Joan Borysenko has talked about "New Age Guilt" . . . a belief that cancer is "because of something." Sometimes cancer just "is" and there's nothing spiritually related to why or where or who or when or how advanced it is. It just exists.

—Z.B., breast cancer survivor

Who knows why I got cancer? What matters now is that I live on. You can help people like me continue living peacefully by not postulating and especially by not sharing theories with us about why we got cancer. We may have already plumbed our souls for the answer. We may have decided that it's simply fate—in fact a recent survey of more than two thousand cancer survivors in the United Kingdom showed that 34 percent believe that cancer occurs by fate—and telling us otherwise may inspire guilt and undermine our healthy hope.

As therapists Pat Fobair, Marty Marder, and Sheila Slattery wrote in "Resilience, A Patient's Perspective" for the Cancer Supportive Survivorship website, 'We don't blame our pets when they get cancer. Why do we blame ourselves?"

"You can't help but wonder, 'Why did this thing happen'?" said Dr. Holland, "Why did the earthquake hit my house and not another one? Why did the disease hit my grandson? Why, why, why, why, why? There isn't any answer and if you go there, it doesn't lead you anywhere good."

You can help us live by leading us to the good places—and by staying there with us.

18.

"Don't take it personally if I don't return your call or want to see you."

Selfishness is not living as one wishes to live,
it is asking others to live as one wishes to live.

—Oscar Wilde

ELIZABETH CARRIED HERSELF with the poise of Carmen Miranda balancing a basket of tropical fruit on her head. The black leotards and white Lycra sleeveless top she donned for her step-aerobics classes revealed a miraculously smooth, flat belly for a woman in her forties who'd given birth to twins.

I walked into her class for the first time, shy and scared. Frumpy in a large black T-shirt, I set up my teal plastic platform in the back of the mirrored room. This was Advanced Step, and I had been stepping only three months. Elizabeth was a dancer whose creatively choreographed step routines changed weekly and challenged her students to move quickly and unconsciously. You almost had to let your body take over; if you let your mind anticipate your moves, you'd get lost.

I credit Elizabeth with helping me live, years before my cancer diagnosis. Stressed and depressed, my system was on overload, and Elizabeth's step routines helped me drop thirty pounds, lower my cholesterol and stress, and ratchet up my self-esteem. But that couldn't keep cancer at bay. When I learned I had the disease, I went to the club to put my membership on hold, because it would be months before I could step again. I ran into Elizabeth.

"I have cancer," I said. She cocked her head a little and lowered her chin. "That's shitty!" she said, a crease forming between her indigo eyes. I was thrilled, not to hear a curse word come from such a sweet mouth, but to know that she truly cared.

"How are you doing with it?" she asked, and I told her about my terror and confusion. She looked at me lovingly, not condescendingly; and as she nodded knowingly, took my hand into hers.

Once I recovered from my surgery, I returned to the club, only to find that Elizabeth was leaving. An ankle injury she sustained as a dancer had worsened, and she could no longer teach. I videoed her last class sometime in May and interviewed her students, some who had climbed hundreds of miles of steps with her during the last fifteen years. Everyone signed an oversized greeting card, and I sent that along with the video to her home. I didn't hear from her that summer and assumed that, as a mother of two youngsters, she was overwhelmed. Neglecting to acknowledge a gift is understandable when you're raising children—especially when they're out of school—so I gave her a pass. But her lack of manners didn't seem to fit with her character.

When I got a letter from her the next fall, it all made sense, in a most disturbing way.

"I'm so sorry I never wrote to you, I meant to, a hundred times," she wrote. "But I was diagnosed with breast cancer, and it has been a whirlwind. You know."

I immediately dialed her number.

"That's shitty!" I said when she answered.

"Well, you know what it's like."

"What can I bring you?"

"How about yourself?" she asked.

> *Don't take what I say personally. It's most likely the drugs that are making me say what I am. If I'm being a bitch, don't bitch.*
>
> —C.T., lung cancer survivor

"Let's go sit by the pool," she said, leading me though a hallway filled with family photos beaming halogen-bright smiles. As the conversation turned to cancer talk, I told her about this book. Her response was like that of most other survivors.

"Do I have a story for you!" Like war stories, survivors often recount cancer horror stories proudly and fondly, nightmarish as they are.

"I have this friend in the Northwest, Adrienne" she began. "She's brilliant; a lawyer. Big cases. Huge heart. So I'm diagnosed with cancer, and my husband and I send an email out to all our friends to let them know. Then we start with all the tests, X-rays, you know the drill." Indeed I did.

"Adrienne calls and leaves me a message on our phone machine," Elizabeth continued, "saying she hopes I'm okay and I should call her. I'm so overwhelmed with what's happening to me and what's going to happen to me, and with my family, that at the end of the day I'm so exhausted I can't remember which toothbrush is mine."

> *I wanted people to understand that I was tired and couldn't return all calls or emails.*
>
> —F.P., breast cancer survivor

Adrienne called again a couple of days later. Elizabeth said she couldn't even remember receiving that message. Then she called again. "This time she leaves me a different kind of message: She says, 'Hey, Elizabeth, what's going on? Why aren't you calling me back? I'm worried. Give me a call. I need to hear how you're doing!'

"I meant to call Adrienne back that night," Elizabeth explained, "but my nine-year-old comes home with poison oak. . . ."

She rolled her eyes. "The next day Adrienne calls again, and she leaves another message on my machine. She says, 'Elizabeth, my husband says I'm just being a selfish bitch, but I really need you to call me'!"

"She was being a selfish bitch!" I agreed. "This is not supposed to be about her! When you have cancer, it's supposed to be about *you*."

I wish I could have said that to my father's friend Danny.

召召召

A most astounding story

When my dad was forty-five, people thought him a decade younger. Even at seventy-five, as he bounced around like the balls he still lobbed on tennis courts, his tanned skin and full head of hair made him look sixty. But by the time he was hospitalized from a fall that led to the discovery of pneumonia, which led four days later to a diagnosis of leukemia, Dad looked every bit eighty-three.

Handsome, even dashing, Dad always took pride in his appearance. He offered to share his "Just for Men" hair dye with my husband, David, whose new beard had grown in silver on his chin and lower cheeks. "Use this and no one will know!" said Dad in loud whisper, like he was sharing a closely guarded secret shrouded in danger. "I've been using it on my moustache for years!"

So it was no surprise that when Dad fell ill in early June 2010, he would not want his friends to see him in the hospital. It wasn't just vanity or pride: his disease weakened him, and he suffered excruciating pain from a condition he developed in the hospital unrelated to his cancer.

"I don't want any visitors," he told me in a tone that warned me not to question his decision. "I'll tell them at the nurses station," I assured him, "and I'll make a sign and put it on the door," which I did, in big black letters highlighted in yellow.

When one of Dad's dear and oldest friends, a woman he dated forty years ago, walked in unannounced and uninvited through the wide hospital room door, I saw embarrassment register on his face, which would have normally lit up like neon. Lying on his back, trapped in bed by tethering tubes, Dad was clearly upset.

"Hi, Norman," said Sandy in a raspy voice. "How are you?"

"Not so good," Dad replied, and within thirty seconds, before I could ask her to leave, he said, "I'm pretty tired, so I'm going to have to go back to sleep."

Although he only wanted to see close family while he was in the hospital, he relented when one friend, Danny, who now lived across the country, said he wanted to come. Dad and Danny's friendship dated back to the 1970s when, as divorced bachelors, they double dated and cavorted in St. Louis's tony Central West End. They continued to talk frequently and double date. Sometimes they vacationed together.

But after passing blood clots for days—the pain Dad experienced was due to the insertion of a urinary catheter that was accidentally yanked out, macerating his bladder—Dad asked us to call Danny and have him reschedule his trip. About a week later, we asked Danny to postpone his flight again, per Dad's request, explaining that he had a horrible reaction to Benadryl.

Finally, when we took Dad home on hospice and Danny once again rebooked his flight to St. Louis, we had to again dis-invite him, per Dad's request. "I don't have time for niceties," Dad had said in the hospital. Now he had much less time, and wanted to save it and the tiny reserve of energy that remained for those he loved most: his wife, Judy; his son, Ron; me, and our families.

 secsec

Dad loved life and laughter more than anyone I have ever known, and although he believed in God (not formal worship, however: "God's so smart he knows that if you thank him once you don't have to go to church to do it every week," he said), he didn't want a funeral. He wanted not tears, but laughs when we thought of him. So we had a life-celebration party and memorial and called it, "It's Been Fun . . . ," named for the autobiography Dad had completed six months earlier.

Danny didn't come this time.

Judy called Danny several times after Dad's life celebration regarding plans they had made together. Danny didn't call back, so Judy finally emailed him: "There are some things I would like to talk to you about as well as catch up on how you are doing."

His response: "Judy, I'm still very sorry that Norman is gone and don't think I have anything more to say. If and when I ever come to St. Louis—I probably won't call you. Sorry, you and your family insulted me in blocking my desire to visit Norman before his death. No further word required or desired from you or anybody in his family. Best regards to all friends of Norman (sic) not including family."

Judy responded to him, and copied my brother and me on the email, excerpted here:

"I feel very sad. I am very sorry you feel that way about the family and me. I hope that you will change your mind. I've been very hurt that you wouldn't talk to me. In fact, I've been crying about it and have tears in my eyes right now as I write to you. It isn't true. We didn't block you from seeing

Norman. It was a nightmare and up and down roller coaster and we were passing on to you what Norman was saying. He kept trying to call you from the hospital. Either he was in pain, horrible pain, or with doctors or the hospital didn't take calls past a certain hour or he couldn't handle the dialing when I wasn't there. He sure didn't want anyone to see him in the hospital. I believe it was his pride. In fact, I felt he wanted to keep his image of the humorous loving person he was. You know it was a nightmare and how up and down it was because you made three attempts to fly in to see him. If Norman were here, he would tell you that I am not the kind of person who would block your seeing him—and would do everything for Norman that he wanted me to do. Please change your mind. I would love to stay your friend (and your wife's, too)—Judy."

Instead of a compassionate response to a widow's grief and tears, Danny wrote:

"Please drop this issue. I don't want to hear from you or your 'family.' I'm sorry you copied them. Maybe, someday, I might feel like talking to you again. That might be quite a while."

I could only imagine how devastating it was for Judy, a deeply loving, forgiving, and kind person, to read such cruel words. It was bad enough that Danny was unable to respect, understand, and accept my father's needs, but to bring his wife and family into it—to misplace his anger or simply reveal his shameful narcissism in such a thoughtless way—was unconscionable to me.

I thought about it for a long time: should I just let it go and write it off to the crazies that grief and trauma can bring out in people? Should I practice compassion for Danny, who was obviously so deeply hurt that he could not or would not acknowledge the pain he had caused?

About a week later, I bought a greeting card, with a quotation by Ralph Waldo Emerson set in simple serif font on a yolk-yellow background: "What lies before us are tiny matters compared to what lies within us."

One friend did not understand when I told her that I didn't want any phone calls, that I needed time to go inside myself to work through the pain. She was offended. Since she is normally a particularly sensitive person, I was surprised at her reaction. I was also angry that she didn't value my feelings.

—S.W., breast cancer survivor

Inside I wrote:

"Dear Danny,

You were such a great friend to Dad while he was alive. I ask that you please continue to be a great friend to him now by apologizing to the love of his life, Judy. It was not she who kept you from Dad. Nor was it Ron. Nor I. It was Dad himself, who simply did not have the energy or will to see anyone but close family, and asked that others stay away.

Perhaps you will understand this someday. In the meantime, I hope you will find the love and compassion within yourself to realize that Judy deserves and needs support now more than ever. It's what Dad would want from one of his dearest and oldest friends."

Danny never responded. It reminds me of the words of author Carolyn Aird: "If you can't be a good example, then you'll just have to be a horrible warning."

Though my father's suffering and death was a mighty curse, may the lesson that his friend Danny teaches be a blessing for others. Taking someone's else's inability or unwillingness to see you as a personal affront—taking something that is about someone else's dignity, pride, and comfort in their final days—can add grave and lasting insult and unthinkable injury to people already tortured by inconsolable pain.

I had a friend who kept calling and leaving messages asking how I was doing and why I hadn't called back. When I finally did, he asked if he could call me later!

—T.R., prostate cancer survivor

19.

"I need you to offer support to my caregiver, because that helps *me*, too."

Please don't tell me to relax—it's only my
tension that's holding me together.

—Ashleigh Brilliant

THERE WAS A TIME WHEN I had only myself to take care of. And I did a very poor job of it. Producing prime-time television documentaries for an NBC station, I had little time for anything else. Although the topics were *prima facie* depressing, they inspired hope in that they offered solutions to grave problems, such as people with mental illness wandering the streets spewing invectives like bile and teen moms bearing babies they hoped would love them unconditionally.

Ultimately I realized what I needed was to *practice* unconditional love rather than expecting to receive it. "You love your documentary subjects more than you love me," a boyfriend complained. He was right. So I broke up with him and got a dog, whom I could love unconditionally.

"I am a good dog," read the headline of the newspaper column. Griffin, a small German Shepherd mix, had been dumped in a city park with a note attached to his collar explaining that, although he was a good dog, his owners "couldn't take care of me, so they left it up to me to find a home."

The letter, written in pencil on lined notebook paper, was signed "A broken home, a broken heart."

I tracked down the couple who found Griffin. When I saw him romping like a puppy through their grassy back yard, my heart opened like the Red Sea and love rushed through like throngs of Israelites toward freedom. When I stroked his lustrous rabbit-soft coat and smelled the top of his head, I melted.

Adopting Griffin was one of the best things I ever did for myself. I loved walking him each morning, even in the pouring Portland rains. I scrambled to escape from work at lunchtime whenever possible to drive the five miles home for a quick ballgame. And I couldn't wait to come home to an exuberant greeting, followed by the sweet music of crunching kibble.

When friends called and said they were bringing meals over and asked whether Thursday or Friday would be best, I could cry. Not only was it a show of their love and support but also it relieved my wife of yet something else to deal with.

—R.R., rectal cancer survivor

Years later, I moved to the San Francisco Bay area for a position as a senior producer. My work days that summer often lasted as long as the summer light, so I would awaken predawn to drive to the thickly forested Redwood Regional Park, high in the hills, where I would scribble in my journal, while the sun rose and Griffin savored the scent of deer and squirrels.

Griffin definitely helped me live. I was miserable in the job that had taken me hundreds of miles from my best friends and family. Though I was hired to produce documentaries, I was told whom to interview for the company's film about breast cancer, and was directed to focus only on treatment, not cause or prevention. More disturbing, I was directed by one of the funders, a pharmaceutical company that manufactured a leading breast cancer drug, to focus on its remedy. I considered myself an ethical journalist, and being told how to spin or slant my stories was tantamount to treason.

Around the same time, my cousin Barbara told me about a book, *Grace and Grit*, which recounted the story of a woman with breast cancer, Treya Killam Wilber. Written by her husband, philosopher Ken Wilber, the book comprised excerpts from Treya's journals interspersed with his narrative. The difficulty of reading about the couple's harrowing battle was mitigated by the profound love with which Wilber wrote the book.

Toward the end of the summer, as I was sometimes traveling to the East Coast for my job and working twelve-hour days while on the West Coast, Griffin began scratching on the door of the room that confined him during the day. (The woman from whom I rented asked I keep him in my bedroom.) It struck me as unfair, unhealthy, and unkind to continue living this way—both for Griffin and me. That, and the pressure from the documentary sponsors spurred me to plan my resignation. On a late September morning over breakfast in an elegant Washington, DC, restaurant, I said to the company president, "I'm sorry, but I can't do this anymore."

I moved into a less expensive home, and just a few weeks later, accompanied my cousin Barbara and her husband, Eddie, to have a lump in her breast biopsied.

"I have cancer," she said, emerging in a wheelchair after the procedure.

Because I had broken out of my career prison, I was free to offer my support to Barbara in a way that would have otherwise proved impossible. Seen another way, because I had taken care of myself, I could now take care of Barbara. And I could better care for Griffin, who had helped me love and therefore truly live again.

Further, because I had just read *Grace and Grit*, I saw cancer in a whole new way. But I never imagined I would encounter Ken and Treya almost a decade later, under entirely different circumstances.

When the student is ready, the teacher will appear

I had just begun conducting research for this book, and was poring through the tall putty-colored file cabinets at the Women's Cancer Resource Center. I lifted out a folder labeled "Caregivers" and leafed through the brochures, articles, and pamphlets. One of the articles jogged my memory: "What Kind of Help Really Helps? by Treya Killam Wilber." It was excerpted from *Grace and Grit*, the book I had read almost a decade earlier.

Rereading the piece was both encouraging and discouraging. It contained almost everything I wanted to share in my book. And it was beautifully written. Treya's descriptions of what helped and hurt were straightforward but gentle. It was so on-target, in fact, that I questioned my own foray into the subject. But a careful rereading of the chapter, particularly the section about being asked about the cause of our cancer, reminded me why I had undertaken this project.

"Why' questions usually lead to feelings of guilt and self-blame, to regrets about the past," wrote Treya, ". . . to fierce resolutions about the future that may be difficult to keep and only lead to guilt when broken. . . . People sensitive to the complexity of the situation might ask a more helpful question, something like, 'How are you choosing to use this cancer?' For me this question is exciting; it helps me look at what I can do now, helps me feel empowered and supported and challenged in a positive way. . . . In our Judeo-Christian culture, with its pervasive emphasis on sin and guilt, illness is too easily seen as punishment for wrongdoing. I prefer a more Buddhist approach where everything that happens is taken as an opportunity to increase compassion, to serve others."

I realized that my cancer had given me the opportunity to share Treya's evergreen message with a new audience [the original book was published in 1991; a second edition came out ten years later], and to share my own stories and those of others. What I didn't realize was that I would also be given the opportunity to share her husband's wisdom, too.

It was at the Cancer at the Turning Point conference in San Rafael, California, that I rediscovered Ken Wilber in an article he wrote for the *Journal of Transpersonal Psychology*. A stack of the reprinted eighteen-page article stood a foot high on one of the tables, amid other cancer information. Though printed in black on white paper, "On Being a Support Person" jumped out from among the brightly colored flyers, booklets, and pamphlets surrounding it. I grabbed the article, and moved slowly toward the door to find a place to read, undisturbed, outside.

The article began: "For almost five years now my wife, Treya, has been battling cancer and for five years I have been serving—sometimes well, sometimes not—as primary support person for her."

What followed was the grit I loved in *Grace and Grit*. It told, with warmth and humor, the no-holds-barred truth of the sometimes hideous reality of caregiving. Mr. Wilber and the *Journal of Transpersonal Psychology* kindly granted me permission to reprint parts of his article.

"As far as support people go, a particularly insidious problem begins to set in after about two or three months of caregiving. It is, after all, comparatively easy to deal with the outer, physical, and obvious aspects of caregiving. You rearrange your work schedule; you get used to cooking, washing, housecleaning or whatever it is that you as a support person have to do to physically take care of the loved one. . . . This can be fairly difficult, but the solutions are also fairly obvious—you either do the extra work or arrange for someone else to do it.

"What is more difficult for the support person, however, and more insidious, is the inner turmoil that starts to accumulate on the emotional and psychological levels. This turmoil has two sides, one private and one public. On the private side, you start to realize that, no matter how many problems you personally might have, they all pale in comparison to the loved one who has cancer or some other life-threatening disease. So for weeks and months you simply stop talking about your problems. . . . You don't want to upset the loved one; you don't want to make it worse for them; and besides, in your own mind you keep saying, 'Well, at least I don't have cancer, my own problems can't be so bad.'"

> *When I had cancer, one of my friends would take my husband out for spicy meals. Keeping him healthy and happy was a definite key to success.*
>
> —A.S., cervical cancer survivor

Wilber explained that the caregiver begins to realize that his or her problems, though minor in comparison to cancer, nonetheless persist and even worsen because now two problems exist: the original one plus the fact that you can't express and therefore solve the original problem.

"The problems magnify; you clamp the lid down harder; they push back with renewed strength. You start getting slightly weird. If you're introverted, you start getting little twitches; shortness of breath; anxieties start creeping up; you laugh too loud; you have an extra drink. . . . If you're introverted, there are times you want to die; if extroverted, times you want the loved one to die. . . . In any event, death hangs in the air; and anger, resentment, and bitterness inexorably creep up, along with terrible guilt about having any of those dark feelings."

Wilber then wrote that the only solution is to talk about those feelings. He mentions support groups and psychotherapy, but warns that the average person (including him) often waits to avail him or herself of such services until "rather late in the game." Typically, most caregivers do what's most understandable, which is talk to friends, families, or associates. But that only helps for a while.

"I may come to you with a problem; I want to talk, I want some advice, I want some consolation. We talk, you are very helpful, kind, and understanding.

I feel better; you feel useful. But the next day, my loved one still has cancer; the situation is not fundamentally better at all. In fact, it might be worse. . . . Later, I happen to meet you again, and you ask how I'm doing. If I tell the truth, I say I feel awful. So we talk. You are again very helpful, kind, and understanding, and I feel better . . . until the next day, when she still has cancer and nothing is really better.

"Sooner or later you find out that almost everybody not actually faced with this problem on a day-to-day basis starts to find it boring or annoying if you keep talking about it. All but your most committed friends start subtly avoiding you, because cancer always hangs over the horizon as a dark cloud, ready to rain on any parade."

Wilber explained how he coped with the aid of support groups, psychotherapy, couples' counseling, and humor. It was almost too late.

I wanted a friend or two of my spouse's to take him out for a drink, as I knew that he needed support—especially the second time around.

—R.C., bilateral breast cancer survivor

"The most difficult emotional problems I had to deal with as a support person were resentment and self-pity. For about a full year, I had a great deal of hatred and bitterness about the situation I was in. I had greatly curtailed or given up editorships at four different publishing concerns. . . . Worse yet, I had given up writing, which I considered my life blood. You simply can't be a full-time support person and carry on a full-time career at the same time. I can't, anyway. . . . If I couldn't write, I saw no particular reason to carry on. Camus said the only really important philosophical question was whether or not to kill yourself. To be or not to be, that is the question. While contemplating this, I drank a lot of beer."

Wilber continued to care for his wife, realizing it was a choice he made of his own free will.

"So each day I reaffirm my choice. Every day I choose once again. This stops blame from piling up and slows the accumulation of pity or guilt. It's a simple point, but actually applying even the simplest points in real life is usually difficult."

Wilber went on to share coping strategies, which for him included making time to write, meditate, and engage in other activities involving self-care, concluding:

"I still bitch and moan, I still get angry, I still blame circumstances, and Treya and I still half-kid (half-not) about holding hands, jumping off the bridge, and putting an end to this whole joke (fortunately, we're both cowards).

And all in all, I'd rather be writing."

⊐⊐⊐

Caregiving can take a tremendous toll on the body as well as the spirit. According to the American Medical Association, "The research literature is replete with findings that family caregivers face inevitable stresses and burdens [that] place caregivers at risk for psychological and physical problems." And the Family Caregiver Alliance writes, "Studies demonstrate that caregivers have diminished immune response, which leads to frequent infection and increased risk of cancers. For example, caregivers have a 23 percent higher level of stress hormones and a 15 percent lower level of antibody responses. Caregivers also suffer from slower wound healing."

A recent study by cancer nurse Katarina Sjövall from Lund University in Sweden showed that in the year after their spouse or partner's cancer diagnosis, people who are married to or cohabiting with a cancer patient suffer 25 percent more illness, including cardiovascular disease, musculoskeletal diseases, abdominal diseases, and depression. And a survey by Navigating Cancer of three hundred twenty-six unpaid caregivers revealed that more than half the caregivers said their health was negatively affected by caring for a loved one with cancer.

What happens when a caregiver falls ill? Not only he or she suffers but the patient as well. If you are a family caregiver and cannot make time for or justify your own self-care, do it for the person you love. Find what soothes and renews you and make a commitment to practice it, be it hot bath, a tennis game, meditation, or flower arranging. Find encouragement to do so through support from other caregivers, whether online, over the phone, or in person.

And if you have a friend or colleague with cancer who has a spouse, partner, or other family caregiver, don't forget them. When an individual has cancer, it's as if the whole family has it. A motto of the Well Spouse Association, a nonprofit spousal caregiving support organization, in fact is, "When one is sick, two need help." A spouse may need support as much as the patient, and the patient will likely be deeply appreciative.

In the lap of love

Dr. Jeff Kane said that a friend who developed a support program for care-givers, and who was also a caregiver, described them as "the patient's uncast shadow."

When I had cancer, my husband, David, was my uncast shadow, caring for me perfectly, daily serving me warmth, compassion, and a listening ear as deliciously healing as bowls of homemade chicken soup. He carried the load of our family: insisted on carrying the laundry up and down the stairs for months after my surgery, paid the bills, and cared for our teen-aged son and four animals.

One of my biggest fears was that David would burn out. Because of the support of his employer, friends, and family, he was able to cope. But my hope and my prayer is that, should I get sick again, he will avail himself of any and all resources to shore up his spirit and give voice to his own pain—that he will take care of himself and enlist the help of others. And that others will unselfishly offer their support.

When I went to the hospital, my daughter was there almost round the clock. But I worried that she wasn't exercising, and I wasn't strong enough to argue with her about it.

—E.C., lung cancer survivor

20.

"I don't know if I'm cured, and bringing up my health can bring me down."

If a man will begin with certainties, he shall end in doubts;
but if he will be content to begin with doubts,
he shall end in certainties.

—Francis Bacon

WITH JUST ONE YEAR TO GO before graduation from UC Berkeley, Terry Healey, a handsome, healthy hunk who headed his fraternity, noticed what he thought was a pimple behind his right nostril. It took five weeks to determine that the lump was not a benign sign of stress known by many an undergrad, but a fibrosarcoma, a rare cancer about which relatively little is known. His tumor was excised, and he needed neither chemo nor radiation, but just a memory zap to forget those surreal two months. A small scar on his nose that made him look like he'd been in fisticuffs was the only reminder—until six months later, when he felt a tingling in his cheek, caused by another malignant mass.

Terry learned he would require extensive surgery, which would result in the loss of part of his nose and cheek, and other parts of his face. During the next six years, he underwent more than thirty reconstructive surgeries to reform his face, almost half of which was removed. He endured other challenges, to his psyche and ego.

"People would actually come up to me when I was riding BART (the Bay Area's rapid transit train system) and ask me what happened to my face."

He never quite got used to the strange and sometimes cruel questions. One time he was sitting at a bar and an older man bellied up and asked, "What in the hell happened to you?"

"I made a judgment that he was drunk and that he would not want to hear the truth," Terry laughed, "So I proceeded to tell him that I had been a DEA (Drug Enforcement Agency) agent who was working with border patrol agents in Texas, monitoring and surveying drug runners coming across the border. 'Out of nowhere there was gunshot,' I told him, 'and a bullet pierced through my cheek and nose'!"

Terry continued weaving the yarn, saying he had resigned from the agency to have his nose reconstructed. The man's response disarmed him.

"He thought I was a hero. He thought that I was everything that America stood for and said he admired me and I was courageous."

Although Terry started to feel guilty about lying, he was too far along to stop. "The guy was eating it up. I'm sure he told all his buddies about me because he was fascinated by it, and we ended up talking for a long time.

Ultimately that experience taught Terry to answer such questions honestly. "That's the only way that people can learn from all these things. So today I make a conscious effort to tell children and adults exactly what happened to me so that they hear the truth from the outset."

"Oh, I just know that you're going to be cured!" That was the worst! I didn't know that at all. Of course I hoped for it. Disease and dying is a part of life for everyone. While I wanted people to be helpful (I did need help), I wanted to deal with the situation as clearly and calmly as possible.

—D.P., cervical cancer survivor

Terry has told the entire truth in a compelling book, *At Face Value: My Triumph Over a Disfiguring Cancer*. He also speaks to groups throughout the nation and often appears in news media. Although it's been more than twenty years since his diagnosis, he is still asked and bothered by the question "Are you cured?"

During a radio station interview, the host asked, "What are the odds of your being cured? Is there a strong likelihood it won't come back?"

Terry said he never asked that question of his doctors, never wanted to know. No two types of fibrosarcoma are alike, so the question didn't make sense to him. "How are you supposed to respond to that?" Terry asked of the interviewer's query. "To me that was never important and it shouldn't be. And doctors shouldn't offer that information up to patients. If I had been told when I was first diagnosed what I know now, I may have not behaved the same way. I was very impressionable."

Telling patients they suffer from an incurable disease can be devastating and, as discussed earlier, may become a self-fulfilling prophecy. And asking if they are cured is something they cannot know. If they believe they are cured, they will tell you that. And if you love them, you will not question that.

Here's the worst: "So you're cured now?" What you want to say is, "No, I have cancer for the rest of my life."

—E.K., lymphoma survivor

"Physician, heal thyself"

Physician Ralph Berberich cured many children in his career as a pediatric hematologist. He felt fulfilled, but after years of working with seriously ill children, he jumped at the chance to join a friend in establishing a new general pediatric practice. After fighting so many cases of cancer, he was relieved to fight the common cold and other relatively minor ailments.

Although Berberich thought he was finished battling cancer, twenty years later, it appeared in his own body. He wrote about it in the book, *Hit Below the Belt: Facing Up to Prostate Cancer.*

"The full impact of treatment goes well beyond facts," he wrote. "It is one thing to read about loss of hair. It's another to see your pubic hair thin to a point you haven't known since before you began adolescence, to see it almost gone. . . . It's one thing to read that you may lose sexual interest, and it is another to walk down the street, see a gorgeous woman, and have your mind register familiar sexual attraction but only in theory. . . . How can books dealing with the facts of prostate cancer truly relate such sensations?"

Hit Below the Belt does so beautifully. It also describes what it's like to be asked whether you are cured of your cancer.

"People meet me today and ask whether I have completed treatment. I tell them that I have. They then often ask, 'Are you cured?' or 'Does this mean the cancer is gone?' No questions could be stranger when applied to cancer in general and to prostate cancer in particular. To most laymen, the word 'cure' means the illness is over for good. Cancer is never really over unless you die, have an autopsy, and are shown to be cancer free, in which case it is of no interest to you. The passage of time simply reduces the chance of recurrence, but it never completely eliminates it."

I can never know whether I'm cured

When someone asks me whether I'm cured, I usually answer, "As far as I know. As far as any of us know, we're cancer-free until we find out otherwise."

I don't say that to disturb the questioner or to intimate that an undetected tumor could be growing stealthily within his body, but to acknowledge that none of us can positively know, at least for now, whether we have cancer (although a new blood test so sensitive that it can spot a single cancer cell among a billion healthy ones is being tested, as is a $200 smartphone device that correctly determined the difference between malignant and benign tissue in 96 percent of cases).

> On the "Are you cured now?" issue, every time they ask it, it drives home the point deep inside of you that you will never know.
>
> –K.G., lung cancer survivor

Some survivors fear declaring themselves "cured" because they're superstitious and don't want to jinx their fate. A recent study published in *Psychological Science* shows that people are more likely to be superstitious during times of uncertainty, when they are under stress and have little control. Some of us knock on wood or perform other reflexive actions to shield ourselves and give ourselves a sense of control. Superstitions such as knocking on wood are a way we abdicate control, while still feeling in control.

"We look for signs, and it's natural because we have stopped living in the ordered logical universe in which there is real causality in our daily lives," explained therapist Halina Irving. "One of the reasons we look for how to control the disease, is that we want the control, but another reason is that as human beings we come into the world with a need to find meaning, reason, cause, and effect in order to be able to live a predictable rational life.

"When you are diagnosed with cancer," Irving continued, "you say, 'But I never ate fat and I never smoked and there's no family history of cancer and I'm such a good person, why did this happen to me?' That world has been then turned upside down for us and that leaves room for superstition."

᠎᠎᠎

We also look to science and seek truth from those trained in the sciences. I don't know a single patient who does not love to hear a medical professional declare her cured. Doctor's words wield tremendous and sometimes even seemingly magical power. I'll never forget the day when the head of pulmonology at the University of California, San Francisco, Dr. David Jablons, indicated I was cancer-free.

"Lori, I believe you are cured of your cancer," he declared. (Dr. Jablons was not my surgeon, but I consulted him for a second opinion, which I believe everyone should seek.) I knew the grim survival statistics for lung cancer, and loved hearing such an esteemed surgeon's judgment, which sounded like a "not guilty" verdict to one who feared she was facing the gallows. Though it did not mean I was cured, it bolstered my hope.

> *When people ask if I'm cured,*
> *I feel like a liar if I say, "Yes."*
> *How do I really know? How does*
> *anyone know?*
>
> —T.E., breast cancer survivor

Even now, almost nine years after Dr. Jablons declared me cured, when I have a "scanxiety" attack or see a frightening cancer headline, I replay his words in my mind and remind myself that I will likely live to play with my son's children and maybe even spend my retirement savings. But I know that Dr. Jablons doesn't have what Dr. LeShan called "a Golden telephone to God." No one knows how much time they have.

How you can help me live

I don't know if I am cured of my cancer, and I do not want you to ask me. I'd rather you not ask me about my health at all. Instead, ask me, "What's up?" If we are close enough, I will bring up the issue of my health. I will bring up my fears—if I feel safe enough to do so.

Take me, Terry Healey, and Ralph Berberich at face value. If we sport a genuine smile, you can assume we are feeling well or "cured," or that we have at least forgotten we had anything to be cured of.

I know the subtitle lists 20 things people with cancer want you to know, but there's one more thing I wanted to add to this edition . . .

21.

"I am more grateful than I can say for your care, compassion, and support."

Gratitude is the memory of the heart.

—Jean Baptiste Massieu

THE DAY AFTER I WAS DIAGNOSED with cancer, I dispatched a mass message to my friends, family, and even colleagues and casual contacts asking them to pray for me or keep me in their thoughts. Within minutes, it was as if a water hydrant cap had blown: loving words and gifts rushed forth, arriving via cyberspace, telephone, and the mail. Plants and flowers, wine and cheese, candles and incense, stuffed animals, novels, gift and healing books, CDs, stationery, other tokens of caring large and small, especially greeting cards—the number one form of social support women with cancer say they like to receive—found their way to my home in the coming weeks.

While recovering from my surgery, I awakened every four hours to take medication that allowed me to stay ahead of the pain from the near foot-long incision that cut through skin, muscle, and nerves to remove a lobe of my lung. I couldn't just grab and gulp the pill, but had to down it along with food, usually a banana. So I took advantage of this opportunity of awakening to let those who had gifted me know how much their gifts—and they—meant to me, creating a nightly, or rather "middle of the nightly," ritual of penning thank you notes.

At first, writing the notes was simply a means to an end. Although I enjoyed the endorphin rush of drawing lines through my friends' names on the list, usually three per night, it was still a duty drilled into me as a child. But soon the ritual became an end in itself. As Herman Hesse taught in *Journey to the East*, the end of the journey was indeed the journey itself. Expressing my thanks was no longer a chore but a practice in gratitude, a practice in focusing on all I had rather than all I lacked or had lost.

Thanking my dear friends, family, and colleagues—Dad and Judy, Marjie and Wayne, Barbara, Alice, Ellice, Lorrie, Ron, Suzy, Amy, Sam, Jordan, Heidi, Cindy, JoEllen, Dale, Alma, Roxanne, Sharon, Kymberli, Peter and Jean, Roseanne, Lizzie, Nasus, the good people of Give Something Back Office Supplies, and so many others—helped me heal. And I believe, to this day, they all helped me live.

I was a single mother, in the middle of a bad divorce. Friends and school families came and took care of us. Took my daughter to school and sports. Set a website for meals and rides. Literally held my hand in chemo. Kept my dogs when I was in the hospital. Kept my kid when I was in the hospital! They saved my life, and I will be forever grateful. Got a huge karmic debt to repay, and I'm happy to do it!

—L.L., breast cancer survivor

Please forgive us if we forget to thank you

Although I was fortunate to have the opportunity and energy to write those notes, many do not. And there was a time that I did not. During the summer of 2010, when my father was hospitalized for weeks and his wife, Judy, and I and other family members spent each day with him, we came home to fresh, comforting home-cooked meals (not just dishes, but entire meals) delivered by Judy's friends. They arranged to pass off keys so they could place the perishable dishes in the refrigerator and keep the homemade chocolate chip cookies from melting on the balmy porch. Our cousins had a stupendous deli tray delivered. Each meal, delivered with love, was deeply appreciated; without them we probably would have lived on take-out, adding physical heartburn to piercing heartache.

Although I intended to pen a note to each person who helped, I was so depleted during Dad's illness, and even more exhausted afterward, that I blew my cardinal rule of manners as well as the opportunity to revive the gratitude practice. I eventually sent a long, sincere, loving thank you note via email to all who helped, but still feel guilty that I neglected to thank everyone in the way they deserved.

Cancer survivor, comedian, and author Glenn Rockowitz might say, "Balderdash!"—or something bluer. In his humorous and sardonic article for the *Seattle Weekly* titled, "How Not to Cheer Up a Cancer Patient," he wrote the following under the heading, "You're Welcome," about sitting in a young adult cancer support group where a distraught friend was trying to figure out how to finish all his thank you notes for the people who cooked for him while he was recovering from treatment.

Benefits were held for me, both at work and by friends. I was taken aback, touched, and overwhelmed. It's hard to accept help, sometimes, but I am so grateful and appreciative.

—D.C., breast and colon cancer survivor

"I told him that I was pretty sure they'd understand if he chose to blow it off. Seriously. If you cooked for a loved one while they were sick or if you walked their dog or helped clean up . . . with the expectation that a Thank You note would be forthcoming, you should probably take a closer look at your definition of love. Or consider a career in puppy-murdering or nun-punching. Of course what you did was incredible and sweet and loving. Please assume that your lumpy pal is extremely grateful. And not just lazy or thoughtless."

One of the kindest things you can do for survivors is to give them a pass on writing a thank you note. If they're anything like me, they'll likely write one anyway, but just knowing while in such a vulnerable state that you will be forgiven and understood is huge. Mammoth, even.

⊐⊐⊐

As sensitive as people with cancer become to slights, neglect, and horror stories, they are just as overjoyed by thoughtful, kind, considerate words and acts, even ones that noncombatants might consider minor or inconsequential. "I ran into a casual friend who had cancer about a year ago, and he went on and on about how grateful he was for all that I did," said my friend Fran. "Funny thing is, I didn't even think I had done anything. I think I maybe brought him a casserole."

Like a small stone spreading vast ripples, even tiny deeds of kindness can radiate joy, not only through a survivor's heart, mind, and soul but well beyond.

In my survey, the statement "I am more grateful than I can say for your care and concern" ranked second among more than six hundred survivors, just behind "I need to laugh, or just forget about cancer for a while." Why? Because, just as it is our biggest fear that people won't be there for us when we need them most—and when we have cancer, we regress to a state of dependency and thus need people more than ever most—our greatest hope is that they will show up.

Showing up for someone with cancer, and offering comfort and solace, can be vastly rewarding. As therapist Halina Irving said, "It gives us the greatest meaning that we can give to our own lives."

What you may get back, in addition to knowing that you have exercised your power to make a difference and enriched your own life, is the same kind of care and concern should you ever fall ill with cancer or find yourself felled by divorce, a loved one's death, or other trauma. I would never, ever wish such trauma on anyone, but if ever you are lost in terror, grief, or hopelessness, I hope you will be able to mouth these words yourself: "I am more grateful than I can say for your care, compassion, and support."

When my father returned to my home for another visit a few weeks after I recovered from surgery, I asked him to help me secure eight strings of red wrapping ribbon across the wall next to my bed. Together we placed get-well cards over each taut row. Some cards dropped sparkles like angel dust onto the hardwood floor below; some burst forth with colorful bouquets or single calla lily blooms; some spoke love through puppy eyes; one cartoon revealed the flabby gray backside of an old man in a hospital gown. I wanted and needed to remember the love that accompanied those cards, as the notes, calls, and emails diminished.

Two years after my scar and psyche had healed from cancer, those greeting cards remained on my wall. "It's time to take them down and move on," I told myself for the tenth time. But I could not let go of the love represented on each piece of card stock. Finally, my sense of cleanliness won out (have you ever tried to feather-dust greeting cards?), and I made a ritual of reading and removing each piece of love-laden cardstock, placing them into a basket. Which remains in my office today.

And helps me live.

part II:

A Quick Guide to Cancerquette

I FRAMED THE FIRST EDITION of *Help Me Live* largely around stories and first-person statements, because they are personal, they engage people, and they add dimension and color to an issue that is decidedly not black and white. But realizing that not only survivors but also their friends and loved ones may have little time to read through all the stories, and may need to focus on a particular type of cancer or circumstance that relates to their own, I included a relatively lengthy appendix.

But when I was writing the revision, I decided to answer the plea of author, essayist, social commentator, and cancer survivor Christopher Hitchens. In a December 2010 *Vanity Fair* article, "Miss Manners and the Big C," as part of a brilliant series he wrote after being diagnosed with esophageal cancer, he called for "a short handbook of cancer etiquette."

My initial reaction after reading Mr. Hitchens's article was "I've already written the handbook he has called for." But I realized *Help Me Live* could not be described as "short."

So what follows are brief sections, comprising lists culled from survivors, including hundreds who answered my survey; excerpts from other books and articles; opinions and advice from individuals and organizations consulted during my research; essays from men and women who wrote about their experiences expressly for this book; and materials from pamphlets and other media, including social media, websites, and videos.

This guide is designed for easy reference. Though it does not contain a separate section for resources as the original edition of this book did, partly because the list has grown exponentially, a new, comprehensive resource page appears on my website. From there you can access directly the information you need. Visit www.lorihope.com/resources.

It is my hope that this section provides not just everything you need to know about how to help your loved one live, but also the joy and satisfaction in helping someone through perhaps the most violent, terrifying tempest they will ever attempt to navigate.

22.

The 2010/2011 Survey

THE FIRST EDITION OF *Help Me Live* was based in part on an anonymous survey distributed through cancer treatment centers, teaching hospitals, cancer support organizations, and public meeting places such as coffee shops and libraries, and it was also sent out into the world via email and old-fashioned flyers. This was in 2004, the year Facebook was founded, and long before I joined the social networking community, numbered at six million seven years later.

Seventy-seven people responded to the survey; not a large enough sample to deem it scientific, which was not the point, but certainly a sizable enough group to validate what the literature, psychosocial cancer support authorities, and cancer survivors I interviewed indicated. For the second edition, however, I wanted to survey a much larger population, not only to validate the previous findings and determine whether the original statements continued to resonate but also to explore differences among people of more diverse ages, backgrounds, and genders, and consider whether new statements were warranted.

I enlisted the aid and advice of several individuals who reviewed the questions and offered suggestions, including Stuart Hanson from the Center for Applied Local Research in Berkeley, California; Kathy Gurland, MSW, LCSW, of the National Association of Social Workers Communication Network; Jeff Kane, MD, founder of cancer support programs at Sutter and Sierra Nevada Cancer Centers; David Spiegel, MD, psychiatrist, psychosocial cancer support researcher and clinician, and Stanford University Medical School/Department of Psychiatry professor; Kairol Rosenthal, author and young adult cancer advocate; and Heidi Adams of The Lance Armstrong Foundation.

Heeding the advice and incorporating the suggestions, I finalized the survey and distributed it through the Internet, including social media sites, cancer organizations, cancer conferences, email, and my electronic newsletter, *Hope Today.*

It took only a few months to collect not 500 but 634 responses, and more than 2,000 additional comments and stories. I found this remarkable, because the survey comprised twenty questions, five of them open-ended, and could take up to twenty minutes or more to answer, depending on the amount of detail respondents chose to include. Regardless of how long it took each individual to complete the survey (completion was not required, though almost all the respondents did complete it), it required careful thought and for many people, the mining of painful memories.

At one point, I felt a pang of fear that started to ache like regret when I stopped by a small storefront in Guerneville, California, to pick up a survey from a survivor who, a week earlier, said she wanted to fill one out. This wasn't just any survivor; she had lived through two bouts of cancer as well as a stroke. When we first met, she asked what I did for a living, and I told her I was a writer. When she asked what I write about, I told her and she shared that she was a survivor. When I told her about the survey, her round face flushed pink.

"It's been twenty-five years since I finished treatment," she said, "so I might not be able to remember what I needed back then, but I want to give it a try!" She was old-fashioned, she said, and didn't want to answer the survey online, so I left a hard copy with her and promised to pick it up in a week.

The first thing she offered when she saw my eager smile again was not a friendly greeting, but an apology: "I'm so sorry, I just couldn't do it."

"That's okay," I assured her without pause.

"I just couldn't go back there," she explained, shaking her gray curls and dropping her eyes. "I started reading the questions and it made me think about it—it's been so long, but it all came back. . . ."

"I am so sorry," I jumped in, realizing or rather, remembering, that I differ from many survivors more "normal" than I, who would rather return to earth, justifiably so, than keep their psyches in the Cancersphere. For me, recalling the surreal skyscape is therapeutic, a reminder of my good fortune, and helping others is a source of satisfaction.

In any case, I worried that I might be harming survivors who had successfully buried painful memories by asking to unearth them. I also wondered whether the survey was skewed toward individuals who believe this subject important enough to invest in, or who have an ax to grind or an experience that is positive or otherwise exceptional enough to want to share. (This is true, to a certain extent.)

Seeking validation of what I inwardly felt was correct, that the survey was indeed helpful, I decided to check the email address I had provided at the end of the anonymous survey, where respondents could write separately to enter a drawing for free health and healing books as a token of appreciation for their time. I wanted to see if others reacted negatively. The other side of the worry coin I'd tossed in the air landed heads up.

"I don't want to be in the drawing, but I want to say thank you . . . it is therapeutic (even after all these years) to answer these questions," wrote one woman from Dublin, Ireland. "Thank you for the thought-provoking and wonderful survey!" wrote another. Other survivors wrote messages such as these: "I just completed your survey, which I found extremely thought provoking. Thank you for doing this." "I found the questions in your survey really hit the mark." And "Thank you for giving voice to the younger survivors!"

It was reassuring to know that, even if the survey upset a few respondents, most who wrote to me found the experience cathartic and healing, and appreciated the opportunity to help others who would come after them.

In this section, you will find the text of the survey, a presentation of the most significant findings, and a few of the most compelling, heartfelt, humorous, or surprising comments, which also appear throughout part I, in the margins.

The Text of the Survey (For brevity, I am including here only the qualitative questions. In the actual survey, I requested information about age, gender, geography, diagnosis, treatment, staging, and ethnicity.)

After you were diagnosed, what did you like/want/need to hear from friends and loved ones? (Please mark as many as apply.)

❑ I'm so sorry this is happening to you.

❑ Call me if you need anything.

❑ I love you.

❑ I'm here to pick up groceries or run errands for you.

❑ You're going to be just fine, don't worry.

❏ I'm here for you.

❏ Other (Please specify.) _____

If you were working outside the home, what did you like/need/want to hear from your boss and/or coworkers? (Please mark as many as apply.)

❏ Don't worry about work. We'll take care of everything.

❏ We miss you a lot.

❏ We hope you get back to work soon.

❏ Other (Please specify.) _____

After diagnosis, what did you need/like/want your friends, loved ones, or colleagues to do for you?

❏ Visit me.

❏ Run errands for me.

❏ Take my spouse or partner out to provide respite for him/her.

❏ Help with my children or pets.

❏ Take me out to a meal or movie.

❏ Keep up my garden.

❏ Update others on my condition or needs.

❏ Send greeting cards.

❏ Call me.

❏ Email me.

❏ Set up a CarePage or CaringBridge website/online community for me.

❏ Do research for me.

❏ Just sit with me.

❏ Help with housekeeping.

❏ Make meals for me.

❏ Go shopping for me.

❏ Other (Please specify.) _____

*If there was anything you did not want people to do, please explain.
(An example might be stopping by without calling first.)*

_____

_____

_____

_____

_____

*What did you not want/need/like to hear from friends, loved ones, or
colleagues? (Examples might be "You just have to think positively!,"
"You have a good kind of cancer," or in the case of lung cancer, "Did
you smoke?" or melanoma, "Did you sunbathe?" From colleagues, an
example might be "Why do you need another month before coming
back to work?")*

_____

_____

_____

_____

_____

*Has anyone ever said anything to you related to cancer that may have been
meant to help you (or was said without forethought) but instead hurt you?*

❑ Yes

❑ No

❑ Not sure (Please explain.) _____

_____

_____

If so, very briefly, please share

a. what was said _____

b. what was your relationship with the person _____

c. under what circumstances it occurred _____

How did it make you feel? (Please mark as many as apply.)

❏ Angry

❏ Hopeless

❏ Disappointed

❏ Confused

❏ Compassionate

❏ Insulted

❏ Accused

❏ Minimized or dismissed

❏ Upset that it took energy I'd rather save for my healing.

❏ Sad

❏ Other (Please explain.) _____

How did you react? (Please mark as many as apply.)

❏ Surprise

❏ Anger

❏ Laughter

❏ Crying

❏ Other (Please explain.) _____

If you did not share how you felt with the person, why not? (Please mark as many as apply.)

❏ You were afraid he/she wouldn't connect with you again.

❏ You were too shocked to react.

❏ You knew he/she meant no harm.

❏ You didn't think it was a big deal.

❏ You were afraid you'd hurt his/her feelings.

❏ Other (Please explain.) _____

Below are the twenty-plus statements those who have had cancer have said they most want others to know. Please check as many or as few as apply to you, ranking them in order of importance if you'd like (1–5).

__ "It's okay to say or do the 'wrong' thing."

__ "I need to know you're here for me, but if you can't be, you can still show you care."

__ "I like to hear success stories, not horror stories."

__ "I am terrified and need to know you'll forgive me if I snap at you or bite your head off."

__ "I need you to listen to me and let me cry."

__ "Asking my permission can spare me pain."

__ "I need to laugh—or just forget about cancer for a while!"

__ "I need to feel hope, but telling me to think positively can make me feel worse."

__ "I want you to respect my judgment and treatment decisions."

__ "I want compassion, not pity."

__ "Advice may not be what I need, and it can hurt more than help."

__ "I am still me; treat me kindly, not differently."

__ "If you really want to help me, be specific about your offer, or help without asking."

__ "I love being kept in your thoughts or prayers."

__ "Hearing platitudes, how strong I am, or what's good about cancer can trivialize my feelings."

__ "I don't know why I got cancer and hearing your theory may add insult to grave injury."

__ "Don't take it personally if I don't return your call or want to see you."

__ "Give me an opening to talk about cancer, then follow my lead."

__ "It's crucial that people who take care of me take care of themselves, too."

__ "I don't know if I'm cured and bringing up my health can bring me down.

__ "I am more grateful than I can say for your care, compassion, and support."

What kinds of social support were helpful to you in fighting cancer? (Please mark as many as apply.)

❏ Receiving greeting cards

❏ Receiving visits

❏ Receiving phone calls

❏ Receiving emails or CarePage or CaringBridge messages

❏ Spending time with family

❏ Online cancer/healing communities

❏ Online support group

❏ Live support group

❏ Exercising/walking with a friend

❏ Dancing with a friend

❏ Watching a movie at home with a friend

❏ Going to a concert or movie or comedy show with a friend

❏ Attending religious or spiritual gatherings (e.g., church, temple)

❏ Other (Please explain.) _____

If there was just one thing about you that you would like people who haven't had cancer to know, what would that be, or if there is a statement (or statements) that you think others should know about people with cancer, please include here and, if you'd like, explain why.

If there are any stories of specific things friends, loved ones, religious or community groups, or colleagues said or did that helped you or buoyed your spirits, please share them here. You may take as little or as much space as you need.

Key findings and a note about apparent contradictions

What follows are key findings from each multiple-choice question, followed by supporting and additional information from the open-ended questions, and finally, statistical data regarding age, type of cancer, gender, and other information about the respondents. Percentages have been rounded off.

If I had to sum up the findings of this survey in one sentence, I would say, "People with cancer need to know you truly care, which you can demonstrate by listening, being respectful of their feelings, offering specific help and following through."

As you will see in the following subsections, and as you have seen throughout the book, a handful of key messages appear again and again, weaving like sturdy reeds through the statements and stories people with cancer want noncombatants to know. As you have also seen, some of the comments made by survivors seem at odds with those of other survivors. In some cases, two comments made by the very same survivor in the very same sentence may seem contradictory. For example, the same survey respondent said that what he did not want was for people to "pretend I was perfectly okay, or treat me like a complete invalid."

Another person noted that she didn't want others to "be afraid to ask questions about what is going on with her," yet hated all the prying (e.g., "invasive questions—I'll tell you what I want to when I'm ready.")

I see such statements not as contradictory but as attempts to help others find a middle ground:

- Don't ignore or obsess: "Give me an opening to talk about my cancer and then take my lead."

- Don't coddle me or minimize what I'm feeling: "I am still me: treat me kindly, not differently."

Although such statements may seem at odds, in fact they point to the same principles: respect, honor, truly listen. In short, make it about the patient, not you.

As for the real differences between individuals, even they are easily reconciled. For example, one person was annoyed that people would "call and talk to my husband instead of me, as if I was too sick to have a phone conversation," while someone else was bothered by people saying they didn't want to call because they were afraid of bothering the patient. Some people wanted their friends to "hide their tears," while others said, "Cry in front of me." And although many said they wanted specific offers of help, many others appreciated hearing, "Let me know if I can do anything."

How to reconcile these differences? How can you possibly know the right thing to do? How to acknowledge the elephant in the room without either tiptoeing around it or tripping on its massive toes?

Simple, just ask:

- "Would you rather I bring up cancer or should I let you be the one to talk about it?"
- "Is it okay if I cry around you?"
- "I'd like to offer specific ways to help you, but would you rather be the one to suggest ways to help, or not ask for help at all?"

Again, by speaking from the heart, straightforwardly and with kind eyes, we defuse tension and clear the way for honest and compassionate communication. That's what everyone yearns for.

What patients want to hear

The #1 statement people want to hear after being diagnosed with cancer is "I love you" with 69% of respondents saying they liked, wanted, and needed to hear this from friends and loved ones. Second is "I'm here for you" (66%), followed by "I'm here to pick up groceries or run errands for you" (45%). Then came "I'm so sorry this is happening to you" (31%).

Just 10% wanted to hear: "You're going to be just fine, don't worry." As discussed in part I, this statement can minimize or trivialize what the patient faces.

Almost 25% of respondents indicated that they wanted to hear other statements from their friends and loved ones as well, such as:

- "You're in my prayers and/or thoughts."
- "Cancer sucks" (and other expletives).
- "Can I give you a hug?"
- "Vent all you like."
- "I care and will always be here."
- "We are going to fight this together."
- "Let's go out for a drink."

What people working outside the home wanted to hear from their coworkers and/or supervisors

- "Don't worry about work. We'll take care of everything." (68%)
- "We miss you a lot." (40%)
- "We hope you get back to work soon." (26%)

Again, about a quarter of respondents added comments about other helpful statements they heard, such as:

- "Start back slowly."
- "Take the time you need to heal. Work is work. Life is living."
- "Your job is waiting when you are ready, you're irreplaceable."

And I particularly liked this one:

- "I'm sorry I didn't realize the seriousness of your illness prior to diagnosis and was a little hard on you despite the fact that you provided doctor's notes every month to support your modified duties."

This resonated with me because when I was in high school, I suffered an attack of appendicitis that almost killed me because a teacher thought I was faking a stomachache to get out of an oral report. Deeply apologetic, she cowered into my hospital room, and I loved watching her chomp on humble pie!

What people wanted friends, loved ones, or colleagues to do for them

More than anything, people wanted to be visited (57%) or emailed (54%). Then came phone calls or having someone just sit with them (50% for both). Other actions that rated highly were updating others on their conditions or needs (38%); making meals (37%); sending greeting cards (35%); taking them out to a meal or movie (30%); running errands, helping with housekeeping, or helping with children or pets (about 29% each).

More than one-fifth of respondents added other things that they wanted friends, colleagues, or loved ones to do for them. Comments included:

- "Wished someone would have helped kids with homework."
- "Cry with me, laugh with me."
- "Put fights on hold."
- "Help financially with grocery gift cards."
- "Go out with me, like to my kids' soccer game, so I could go and be sure I would be alright."

People who heard comments that were meant to help but instead hurt them

More than two-thirds of respondents said that someone had said something to them related to their cancer that may have been meant to help, but instead hurt them. While 4% weren't sure, the remaining 29% said no.

Interestingly, as the survey conducted in 2004 for the first edition of this book indicated, many of the respondents who answered in the negative to this query, also told stories elsewhere that indicated someone *had* actually said something that wasn't helpful. In the first survey, a respondent with colon cancer who answered "no" here, later listed some annoying remarks she heard, including: "Oh, colon cancer. Don't worry, you'll be okay."

Another "no-sayer" wrote that she only told family and three friends because she was afraid how people would react. Yet another said, "I couldn't deal with hearing about people who died from breast cancer or who had metastases. I did not join a support group because of my fear about hearing 'bad' news about how others were doing."

Another survivor answered the question about whether anyone had done anything to hurt them, "Actually, no, perhaps because I was so open with my cancer. I chose not to keep it a secret, but instead, talked about it openly. Perhaps that made people feel more at ease with the subject and didn't create awkward moments where something hurtful might have been said. I still encountered people who didn't know how to respond, but I tried to put them at ease. Their uncomfortable silence enabled me to talk to them and make them feel less uncomfortable considering the topic of cancer."

In the new survey, a sixty-one-year-old thyroid cancer survivor answered no to this question. But to the question about what she did not want to hear, she responded that a friend had said to her, "Better you than me."

She added that someone said to her mother, "She's so young, with two kids!" And a seventy-six-year-old rectal cancer survivor said what he did not like to hear was "Exaggeration of my condition, which I have felt all along was fortuitously a mild case compared to many people who were far more seriously afflicted."

The difference in this apparent contradiction or denial of feelings might be that the person with cancer was not hurt by the insensitive, inappropriate, or annoying statement. Some people do have thicker skin and are better equipped to defend themselves.

Of those who answered that something unwanted had been said to them, 68% indicated that it made them feel angry; 48% felt minimized or dismissed; 47% felt sad; 44% said they were disappointed; 43% felt insulted; and 27% said they were upset that it took energy they would have rather conserved for their healing. Others felt hopeless, confused, accused, or frightened. A few felt guilty ("for not feeling relieved that it was *just* breast cancer"); "unloved;" "alone;" "DISGUSTED;" and "unheard," among other feelings.

As for how the survivors reacted, 27% were angry, 22% were surprised, 19% cried, and 7% laughed. Some reacted with dismay or a cold silence: "I had no words. I said nothing." One person "faked interest . . . so as not to be rude, at first. Then eventually I got to asking the person how they think that story (a cancer horror story) might actually be of some help to me." Some pretended the offender was right; others "left the scene." One person who, because she "tends to be a pleaser, smiled and agreed. Yet another reason for why it hurt so much. I was angry with myself, too." Other respondents said they reacted with "absolute utter despair;" withdrawal and depression; and "probably passive-aggressive" behavior.

If they did not share how they felt with the offender, it was because they were too shocked (44%) or knew the speaker meant no harm (42%). And 15% feared hurting their friends' feelings, while 9% feared their friends wouldn't contact them again. Just 3% said they didn't react because they didn't think it was a big deal.

Some people (25%) added comments, explaining why they did not share their feelings with the offender. Most said they didn't think it would do any good, or that they didn't want to waste time and energy; one woman said she thought she would start crying; another said, "I was afraid I was going to slap her." Another said, "I was worried she [the offender] was crazy pants." One woman wrote, insightfully, "I knew she was afraid of my diagnosis and could not discuss it with me."

Ranking the 20 statements people with cancer want others to know

The results of the new survey reflect what the original survey found, which is that, more than anything, people with cancer say they need to laugh or just forget about cancer for a while, the number one statement in both surveys. Beyond that, the order of the statements differed slightly, partly because some of the original statements were slightly modified, and two new ones were introduced.

One of the new statements, "I am more grateful than I can say for your care, compassion, and support," ranked second in importance. How reassuring! What this says is that no matter how uncomfortable you might feel, no matter how frightened of saying or doing the "wrong thing," and no matter how long you stay away out of fear or embarrassment, whatever you say, give to or do for your friend or loved one will be deeply appreciated. As stated throughout this book, as sensitive to slights that people with cancer may be, they are just as sensitive to love, gifts, and support.

As in the first survey, wanting to be kept in others' thoughts and prayers ranked among the top three statements. Others in the top ten include:

- "I need you to listen to me and let me cry." (#6)

- "I want compassion, not pity." (#5)

- "I need to feel hope, but telling me to think positively can make me feel worse." (#8)

- "Don't take it personally if I don't return your call or want to see you." (#9)

For the complete ranking of all the statements, please visit my website, www.lorihope.com.

The open-ended questions

We asked five open-ended, qualitative questions in the survey. This was done to elicit further comments and stories, exploring in more depth the needs and desires of people with cancer. It was also designed to further validate the top twenty statements presented in the first edition of the book.

The questions about wanted and unwanted words and actions, and about other statements people with cancer might want others to know, consistently elicited the same types of answers and even the same words.

In the hundreds of comments and stories, words and expressions such as "pity," "feel sorry for," and "sympathy" appeared again and again, 237 times, in fact.

Social support

I added this question to the new survey because I thought it would be useful to understand what kinds of social support are most helpful to people with cancer. This may help you know when and how to show up and show you care.

For 74% of respondents, spending time with family helped them the most, while 70% named greeting cards, followed by visits and phone calls (59% for both). Half of the respondents liked receiving emails, CarePages, or CaringBridge messages; about one-third found attending church helpful, matched by online cancer and healing communities and support groups. Just a little more than 25% liked live support groups, perhaps because, as some of the other comments indicated, it can be frightening and terribly sad to see other group members fare poorly.

Additional forms of support were indicated by 23% in separate comments, such as attending Cancer as a Turning Point conferences; "telephone messages, but not feeling I have to return them;" "having my dogs by my side;" joining an "art group for nonartistic peeps like me;" "Facebook messages and wallposts;" "receiving text messages;" and "being a part of raising awareness and funding for a cure" through participating in fundraising walks and other events.

Ethnicity

This survey was not intended as a comparative tool to examine ethnic and cultural differences in cancer treatment or access, but we nevertheless attempted to reach a diverse group of people, which we did through working with various health and cancer support organizations. We reached out to underserved communities by providing printed surveys and requesting assistance from organizations that target such communities. Ultimately, 87% of the survey respondents were Caucasian, followed by 5% Other/Multiracial, 4% Black/African American, 3% Hispanic, 3% Asian/Pacific Islander, and 2% Native American.

Although you will see in chapter 28 that there may be perceived differences in needs and attitudes of people from different backgrounds, most people seem to have the same psychosocial needs: to feel cared for, respected valued, loved, and heard.

This is reflected in the near-identical survey responses of people of different ethnicities. The multiple-choice questions were consistently and remarkably similar across the board: 67% of all groups said that something had been said to them that hurt them; the gender balance of each group was the same (16% male); the most helpful forms of social support matched almost evenly. Even the twenty statements were almost identically ranked, although the statements about prayer and the need to laugh and forget were flip-flopped in Caucasian vs. other ethnic groups, by a very small percentage.

- All groups listed "I am more grateful than I can say for your kindness and support" as second in importance

- Caucasians named "I need to laugh or just forget about cancer for a while" as the #1 statement.

- "I want to be kept in your thoughts and prayers" was ranked #1 by other groups.

Gender

Of the 526 people who included information about their gender in the survey (interestingly, many did not), 16% were male, and 84% were female. Remarkably—or not so remarkably—many of the answers were marked identically by male and female survivors. We certainly share many more similarities than differences.

The top four statements men and women wanted others to know were ranked the same by both genders:

1. I need to laugh. . . .

2. I am more grateful than I can say. . . .

3. I love being kept in your thoughts or prayers.

4. I am still me; treat me kindly, not differently.

The other sixteen statements were chosen similarly, with two main differences: "I need to feel hope, but telling me to think positively can make me feel worse" was ranked #7 among women, #16 among men. Men seemed more forgiving, ranking "It's okay to say or do the 'wrong' thing" #10, as compared to women's ranking of #15.

Men and women alike chose "I love you" most frequently as the statement they wanted to hear after being diagnosed with cancer. Second was "I'm here for you." The statement both genders marked least often as the one they like to hear was "You're going to be just fine, don't worry." Not surprisingly, men were half as likely to want to hear, "I'm here to pick up groceries or run errands for you."

Males indicated they wanted to hear "I'm so sorry this is happening to you" half as much as women. Not surprising, considering that men are generally more sensitive to rank, and the word "sorry" may connote pity more than sadness. And as Matthew Loscalzo points out (see chapter 27 for a detailed analysis of the different needs of men and women with cancer), men are typically less comfortable with feelings of sadness than anger.

I saw this principle firsthand during a predawn morning cab ride to the airport to board a plane for a speaking engagement. I initiated a chat, as I frequently do, with the driver, who was from Nigeria. He asked what I spoke about, and when I told him I was a cancer survivor who spoke about how to support other survivors, he shared that he had irritable bowel syndrome. I immediately said, "I'm so sorry to hear that," and then thought to ask him if that's the kind of thing he likes to hear when he tells someone about his condition. Without taking a moment to think, he said bitterly, "No. I don't want anyone's pity." Because he was from Africa, I thought perhaps there was not a linguistic or semantic difference between someone being sad that another is hurting and someone feeling pity, so I explained that what I meant by "I'm so sorry" was that I am sorry that he is feeling pain, but that I did not pity or look down on him. "But I don't want to hear about people's sadness," he said. "I want to hear, 'I hope you feel better.'" Another example of our differing needs and the importance of inquiring about your friend or loved one's needs.

Of the 434 women and men who worked outside the home and answered the question regarding what they wanted to hear from their boss or coworkers, 67% of both women and men indicated that they most want to hear "Don't worry about work. We'll take care of everything." But more men (33%) wanted to hear "We hope you get back to work soon" than women (24%).

The most significant difference between females and males was that 70% of women said someone had said something to them related to cancer that hurt them, while only 42% of men did. Again, not surprising, given how much women need and value social support.

Both men and women responded most frequently that the gaffe made them feel angry (68% for both genders). Women were more likely to feel dismissed or minimized (50% to men's 41%); accused (17% to men's 9%); and upset that it took energy they'd rather save for their healing (27% to men's 15%). Women and men said they reacted, first, angrily, in equal proportion. Women were more than twice as likely to cry, and men were more than twice as likely to laugh. When asked why they did not share how they felt with the offender, both men and women said, first, they were too shocked to react, and second, they knew the person meant no harm. Men were more likely to say they didn't say anything because they didn't think it was a big deal.

Both women and men said the kind of social support that was most helpful to them was spending time with family. Men and women ranked visits, phone calls, emails, and CarePages or CaringBridge messages as favorite kinds of support, but women said most often that they liked receiving greeting cards (men liked cards half as much). So friends, colleagues, and loved ones, keep those cards, calls, and messages coming. Just don't expect a thank you or return call. It's not about you now. It gets to be about them. They may be exhausted and overwhelmed.

Location, age, and type of cancer

The 634 individuals who answered the Help Me Live Cancer Support Survey ranged in age from fourteen to eighty-nine; 77% were older than forty, 23% were younger. They hailed from more than a dozen countries, including Scotland, UK, and Australia, and from cities A to Z, (Alcante, Spain to Zanesville, Ohio). Most were from the US, and listed more than 350 different zip codes, and cities large and small, from The Big Apple to little Benton, Kansas.

Respondents listed almost fifty different kinds of cancer. The most common was breast (188) followed by lung (78), blood cancers such as leukemia and lymphoma (72), then gynecologic, gastroenterological, glandular, and skin cancers. Several individuals had rare cancers such as adenoid cystic carcinoma, multiple cancers or complicated diagnoses or misdiagnoses. Many were long-term survivors; one man was diagnosed thirty-four years ago.

23.

Different Kinds of Cancer

ALTHOUGH WE SAY "CANCER" as if it is a single disease, there are more than two hundreds varieties, which differ not only in biology but in their psychosocial impact. Some are more curable or common, some carry more stigma than others. I've chosen to briefly discuss a few kinds of cancer you may want to pay special heed to here. This by no means assigns more importance to them.

Breast cancer

I had two close first cousins who had breast cancer during their thirties and forties, and as I said previously, I thought that gave me an intimate understanding of cancer. But you cannot truly know what it's like to have your body turn against itself until it does, and when it threatens a part of you that is private yet public, precious yet not necessary for life itself, sexual yet not necessary for sexual relations, cancer can become more complicated.

Though all women experience breast cancer differently, it is safe to say that most believe the subject should be treated with extra sensitivity. As Susan Love, MD, surgeon, president of the Dr. Susan Love Research Foundation, and author of what the *New York Times* termed ". . . the bible for women with breast cancer, " told me, "You should never assume that a woman would or wouldn't want a mastectomy. Some women do, and some women don't." Sarah, whom you met in chapter 2, said she didn't give her breasts a thought. "I got them both whacked off," she explained. "When I got diagnosed with cancer, I didn't go through some of the stages other women do."

Many other women, especially younger women, may feel very differently. Best not to offer your opinion unless asked, and even then, consider your audience. If you're a woman, take a moment to think about how you would feel if your breasts were threatened.

Special care should be taken when asking questions and offering other suggestions such as those shared by my some of survey respondents:

"Did your mother have breast cancer?" when I responded, "Yes," the people (this happened at least five times) visibly sighed in relief that there was a reason why I had this."

"[It was unhelpful when] someone suggested I not have reconstructive surgery following my mastectomy so I could make a political statement by having no breast. Also unhelpful was 'There are so many things they can do for breast cancer now.' While it may be true that there are more treatments than before, breast cancer still kills over forty-thousand women in this country per year, plus thousands/millions more all over the world."

"I wanted my husband to say he would love me just as much without a breast and I was still beautiful to him. I did not want people to say things that made me feel sorry for myself."

Prostate cancer

As with any form of cancer, it is important to ask permission before asking personal questions, but in the case of prostate cancer, it is particularly important since, like breast cancer, it can and often does affect a man's sense of his sexuality.

Prostate cancer survivor Jim Kiefert, past board chairman of Us TOO International, a prostate cancer education and support network of three hundred twenty-five support group chapters, wrote: "Men *hate* the words 'impotent' and 'castrate.' ED (Erectile Dysfunction) is better than impotent and castrate makes us pucker. . . . We also don't like 'hormone treatment.' Sounds like we *get* hormones."

Wrote one man after reading my book: "As with women who have had their bodies changed during breast cancer treatment, men, too have less noticeable changes after prostate cancer surgery—probably more psychological than physically apparent. My colleagues—all nurses—didn't check in with me while I was absent from work and didn't really ask me how I was doing after I returned. I think that they felt that I was "surgerized" and that took care of everything. It didn't take care of the emotional and physical aspects of healing and support was hard to come by. My wife chose to play no role in my physical recovery and life just went on as before—without a sexual relationship of any note. Imagine how that would make a man feel."

The following statements from my survey respondents who survived prostate cancer provide additional guidelines:

"I didn't like people telling me their father/uncle/brother had prostate cancer, too, and everything turned out okay—before they found out mine was the bad kind. It was a reminder that I was in the tiny minority."

"I didn't like hearing that my postoperative recovery could be as long as six months to a year. Dealing with incontinence and erectile dysfunction was tough."

"I didn't want to hear the horror stories of someone who had died from prostate cancer. Some people like to revel in the gruesome details. I chose to avoid those kind of people."

Lung cancer

I have never heard of a newly diagnosed lung cancer patient who wants to be asked by anyone other than a health-care provider whether he smokes or has smoked, or who wants to hear that he should quit. Hold your tongue. Don't add insult to injury. Everyone knows smoking is dangerous, and telling someone that can be injurious as well. In fact, a study by the University of Oxford in the United Kingdom showed that the stigma attached to patients with lung cancer can have a serious negative impact on their physical and mental health. The study found the stigma, shame, and blame caused some patients to conceal their illness, which sometimes resulted in their not seeking all the required treatment for their disease.

Up to 20 percent of those diagnosed with lung cancer never smoked. When people ask if we smoked, some lung cancer survivors, including myself, relish the opportunity to enlighten them of that fact. But many cancer survivors do not. Let the survivor bring up the subject. Additional comments from my survey reveal what others want you to know.

"The worst question was 'Did you smoke?' When someone is diagnosed with heart disease, no one asks them if they ate too much fried food!"

"I hated when people said, 'I didn't know you smoked' . . . I had lung cancer and have never smoked in my life!"

"When I was first diagnosed, . . . when we disclosed to my mother-in-law and father-in-law, he said, 'Well, I guess this is a sign that you will finally quit smoking then.'"

Melanoma

Like lung cancer, people with melanoma and other forms of skin cancers often field questions about the cause of their cancer, such as "Did you use sunscreen?" Again, people with cancer want to look forward, not backward, and they don't want to feel blamed or guilty about lifestyle choices they may have made, especially if they were made before the dangers of the choices were understood. Here are other comments from skin cancer survivors who answered my survey:

"Some people are rather dismissive when you tell them you have melanoma. Cancer is cancer, and I wish more people would understand that."

"My first occurrence [of melanoma] was on my scalp. 'Did you spend a lot of time in the sun?' Did you wear a hat? Did you use sunscreen? Do you think your kids will get melanoma?"

Rare cancers

It's important to do research on cancer in general—and your friend's type of rare cancer, in particular—before asking about it. It will help you avoid asking questions that could hurt, such as "Aren't there some clinical trials you could enroll in?" Most rare cancers receive fewer research dollars, and asking about clinical trials can kill hope.

One angiosarcoma survivor said he often fielded the question, "So why don't they cut it out?"

"Because a cancer of the connective tissues, nerves, and blood vessels can't be cut out—it's crabgrass, not a stump," he said. "But that doesn't compute. We have one well-meaning friend who asks that question out of frustration about once every four months."

As one woman with leiomyosarcoma, a quickly mutating cancer, told me, "Friends think since you're having chemo you'll be fine, but no, it only works for a few months. Sometimes you just want to say to them, 'How in the hell do you know?' Basically you know people are trying to be nice, but it can be very hurtful."

Another comment from a woman with granulosa cell tumor: "Someone said to me, 'This is the best cancer you can have! It is going to be okay. No one has ever died from this cancer.' In fact, 80 percent die from it. Very rare cancer."

24.
Cancer through the Stages

ALTHOUGH MOST PEOPLE with cancer share certain needs, their needs may change over time and through treatment. The follow sections offer guidelines and suggestions that may help inform your words and actions.

Soon after diagnosis and before treatment

For many people, the first few days or weeks following diagnosis are the most harrowing. Not only do we experience shock, fury, and terror that most of us have never felt before, but we may feel trapped and immobilized because so much remains unknown and we cannot yet harness our energy toward action. As David Servan-Schreiber, MD, cancer survivor and author of *Anti-Cancer: A New Way of Life*, notes, "Fear paralyzes. That's its nature. When an antelope senses a lion's presence, its nervous system sends out a signal, and it freezes. . . . When we find out our lives are seriously endangered, we often experience this strange paralysis of body and mind."

A true trauma for most people, cancer changes us in ways almost impossible to describe. "It really feels like all at once, from one moment to the next, that we've been plunged into the world of the absurd in which nothing makes sense," said Halina Irving, drawing from her experience as both therapist and two-time cancer survivor. "Something has happened to us that goes against everything we ever believed would ever happen to us."

Irving said that although newbie cancer patients are often told to think positively (and who wouldn't want to?), usually our minds are too muddled to function in an even remotely normal fashion. "That person feels that there's a wild beast chasing them, and how can they think clearly and be proactive and feel positive when they have to escape from the clutches of death?"

We may also feel guilty, angry at our body's betrayal of us, and deeply lonely, and our feelings may be volatile, changing quickly and frequently. We fear not only death but also disability and the loss of independence. We fear the unknown. And because we know relatively so little, incessant and insistent questions can be truly terrifying. It's never a good idea to ask too many questions of cancer patients—much better to let them take the lead and tell you what they would like you to know—but this is especially true of those patients who have just learned that there is a whole curriculum they have yet to tackle.

What do newly diagnosed patients need? Love. Patience. Support. A shoulder. A hand. Reassurance. A listening ear and, as earlier noted, kind eyes. And also what these survey respondents offered:

"Immediately after, I needed quiet time alone to listen to my heart and head (and have one good sob session). Then I just wanted my friends and family to be themselves; supportive but not fawning."

"At this point (two weeks after being diagnosed with Hodgkin's), I don't feel like talking about the disease and while I want my friends and family to know I'll be okay, I'm running out of 'explaining' energy."

During treatment

When I was a medical reporter, I remember once using the term "side effects" when interviewing a doctor about a pharmaceutical treatment. He corrected me, saying something like, "There are not *side* effects, there are *effects*, plain and simple." In other words, a side effect can be like a main dish, an entrée all in itself, not just something on the side. A side effect can exert more power than a treatment itself.

I was fortunate that my only cancer treatment was surgery and I suffered few side effects. (A fellow lung cancer survivor whom I had helped for several years, chided me because I didn't have to go through what she went through—the dark side of cancer: jealousy and schadenfreude.) But most others endure treatments such as chemotherapy and radiation in addition to or in place of surgery, and suffer not only physical but psychological effects that exacerbate the pain or trauma of treatment. I will talk first about surgery and hospitalization and then follow with survey quotes regarding other forms of treatment.

Surgery

When I was younger, the idea of someone cutting into my body did not frighten me much. As a high school freshman facing an imminent emergency appendectomy, my biggest worry was the deforming bikini scar it would leave. But many of us become more leery of surgery as we age. I was terrified of having my ribs split open and a lobe of my lung removed through a foot-long incision.

Books and tapes about preparing for surgery through meditation and visualization calmed me, and I would recommend such resources for anyone anxious about going under the knife. Even though surgery now often means going under a much smaller knife due to the development of robotic technology and video-assisted surgery, it can still be very frightening. You can help assuage fears by reading some the following comments from my survey.

"During my time of surgery, I wanted to hear about quick and easy recoveries . . . great stories about my surgeon . . . how unlikely it was that I would develop lymphedema (painful swelling of the upper arm). . . . Post-op I wanted to hear what great progress I was making and how quickly I was recovering . . . that the pain I was experiencing was normal."

"I liked hearing that it was normal to be so very tired after the surgery, because I could do very little without being exhausted."

"During treatment (surgery in my case), I wanted to hear how well I was doing, how good I looked, how strong I am. I didn't want to hear how skinny I had gotten or how scared they were for me. That just made it worse."

Hospitalization

A friend of mine who was recently diagnosed with cancer almost refused surgery because he had heard so many hospital horror stories even though the feared dangers far outweighed the risks. What I encountered, more than stories about infections or poor nursing care, were tales of uninvited visitors who stayed too long or talked too much. Before you visit, make sure you are welcome. Ask permission.

Patients can find it uncomfortable to ask visitors to leave once they appear, so it's important that you ask how long you should stay. Be sure to emphasize that it won't hurt your feelings if they need you to leave.

If you do visit, try to relax. People who are sick may become more sensitive to movement and stimuli of any kind.

Many patients appreciate flowers and low-maintenance plants, but check to see if they're allowed (they are not in some places). Also ask before bringing books. One friend who was hospitalized for several weeks said she received many more books than she had the time or energy to read, and it made her feel bad because she could not tell the gift-bearers she had read what they had given her.

Other comments from survey respondents include:

"[I liked visitors to] sit, let me sleep in their presence, read to me, tell me the banalities of their life instead of asking me to rehash my violent hospital experience over and over."

"There were times, especially in the hospital, that I felt smothered. People just did not get the clue that I did not need nor want seven people in my room while getting a bone marrow biopsy. I remember one time having six visitors in my room and having to go to the bathroom so bad I was afraid I was going to have an accident. They did not get the hint that I needed them to leave."

Chemotherapy

Many with cancer fear chemotherapy more than any other treatment and sometimes even more than the cancer itself. Although it can preclude further suffering and save lives, chemotherapy may devastate the intestinal tract and stomach by killing normal fast-growing cells as well as cancer cells, causing nausea, vomiting, and hair loss. Other chemotherapeutic agents cause other side effects such as rashes.

I cannot describe what it's like to undergo chemo, but I have been told it is like the worst imaginable flu. What follows are some statements from people who answered my survey:

"What I wanted to hear during chemo was 'We will get you through this!'"

"I appreciated jokes about the chemo (such as calling the bright blue stuff the 7/11 Slurpy Blue Chemo) and any comments about the chemo as helping to fight the cancerous cells."

"During chemo, it hurt to hear, 'It's only hair.'"

"A classmate in the master's program I was in kept insisting that he was going to pull my wig off so that he could see how my head looked. I wanted to slap him."

"I had a long talk with a friend who is a homeopathic practitioner. He kept telling me that the chemo was poison and encouraging me to deny it and try some nontoxic treatments. It didn't help me at all. My choice wasn't respected, and I was left with a sinking suspicion that I may be choosing to poison myself."

"I didn't like it when people were constantly asking me if I had lost my hair. And 'Are you throwing up?' and wanting full details of my nausea."

"Several well-meaning friends told me horror stories about huge weight gains . . . and having to self-inject with meds (in the stomach) and terrible nausea. None of those things happened to me or anyone I met while going through chemo and radiation. EVERYONE is different and reacts differently to the medications."

"I didn't like the comments that trivialized or denied how awful I felt some days right after chemotherapy. I'd hear comments like 'But you look soooo good.' They were meant to be polite, but they just irritated me because comments like that suggested I was somehow lying about how bad I felt; insinuated that if I looked good, I must have felt good, too."

Radiation

Conventional cancer treatments—surgery, chemotherapy, and radiation—have been referred to as slash, poison, and burn. Just as most people going through chemo don't like to hear it called poison, most undergoing radiation don't like to think of it as being burned, and, indeed, it does not always cause a burning sensation; sometimes it saps energy, and other times people experience no negative side effects. Those who answered my survey indicated they appreciated sensitivity, honesty, and openness when they were undergoing radiation:

"The doctors [minimized] the side effects of radiation, even as I was suffering them. 'That will go away' was not helpful. More helpful would have been advice about coping."

"Once I decided to go ahead with radiation, I didn't want to hear stories about how dangerous radiation is or how it causes cancer. I wanted coaching on how to see radiation as a positive thing (think of the radiation as sunlight, shining on your breast and healing it)."

"Unhelpful words: 'Oh, radiation treatment is really no big deal, you'll feel a little tired. . . . I was fatigued for a year and a half after radiation. Every woman's experience is unique, and don't dismiss the serious risk and potential bad outcomes."

"Unhelpful: 'But you look so healthy'—like just because you have your hair and don't look sickly, the radiation is nothing.

Posttreatment

Three months after I completed treatment, had you asked whether I was in remission I might have burst into tears. If you asked to bring a hot meal over, I might also have wept. Still raw from my diagnosis and surgery, still worried about whether and how I could possibly integrate the experience into my life and move on, I felt like I had premenstrual syndrome on steroids. One day I would awaken and shed a few tears of gratitude because I felt so fortunate to be alive; other mornings I'd whimper with uncertainty about what the day might bring.

Those were the days I stayed in bed. Though cancer had taken thirty-five pounds off my frame, my body felt like an anchor, dragging me down, hiding me from the world and the light. My wound had healed, but my soul had not. I could not return to the normal I knew before; it had vaporized. I was depressed. A normal and common effect of cancer, discussed further in this section, the fog of depression often rolls in unnoticed. Like becoming nearsighted, it may happen so slowly you fail to notice until you run into a wall. And you may not feel it at all; upon my diagnosis of depression, I felt numb.

The posttreatment period can hit some people much harder. A 2008 study by the Dana-Farber Cancer Institute, published in the *International Journal of Gynecologic Cancer*, showed that 26 percent of early-stage ovarian cancer survivors who were tested had mental health scores suggestive of posttraumatic stress disorder, or PTSD.

Concerns about recurrence are common among survivors as well. *Facing Forward, Life After Cancer Treatment: A Guide for People Who Were Treated for Cancer*, a booklet published by the National Cancer Institute states, "Worrying about the cancer coming back (recurring) is normal, especially during the first year after treatment. This is one of the most common fears people have after cancer treatment."

Indeed, a form of this has even found a new and catchy name, "Scanxiety," a common term in the lexicon of cancer. It needs no explanation among people facing imminent CT scans or other predictive or diagnostic tests, and if you think about it for a moment, you'll know exactly what it means.

It's vital to be sensitive to such conditions and worries, as well as other posttreatment concerns, but not to bring them to your friend's attention, as the following survey comments indicate:

"I wanted people to ask how I was doing, but not to indicate they were asking about my cancer. Sometimes I was able to forget I had had cancer, and didn't want to be reminded by their acting overly concerned."

"Mostly, after time goes by, after treatments are over, one wishes to find normal life again, and sometimes people don't let you forget, by always acting as if you are fragile."

"No matter how one handles the decision making or treatment, this is a journey—even after the treatment is over, there are continuing checkups, physicals, etc., that bring back the dark times and fears. Lots of things can trigger thoughts of metastasis or recurrence—a poor bone density test, a new pain, a change in cholesterol levels even.

Long-term survivors

During the first year after completing treatment, I did not think I could ever feel normal or go a day without worry about cancer. But, indeed, during the second year, days and weeks passed without my considering the disease at all. Even so, the experience, the memories, and the fears remain and can arise quickly, no matter how many months or years have passed. As the NCI booklet referenced earlier indicates, "Even years after treatment, some events can cause you to become worried about your health. These may include: follow-up visits; anniversary events (like the day you were diagnosed or had surgery or ended treatment); birthdays; illness of a family member; symptoms similar to the ones you had when you found you had cancer; the death of someone who had cancer."

The following comments from the Help Me Live Cancer Support Survey provide other insights:

"Many people [including] friends [and] family have indicated that 'it's over now' since I'm four years postdiagnosis. Well, it's not over, as I still have fear of recurrence, which is near impossible to discuss with anyone outside the Cancer circle.

"I still fear cancer [years later] and it's still got a grip on my emotions. It is hard to share your fears, especially when 'healthy' people can't understand the longevity of them."

"There was a time when I thought I would think about my cancer every day and now, thirteen years later, I don't. But it still intrudes at times and then I'm right back there. So recognize the pain and try to give some quiet hope, but, of course, be careful how you say this."

End-of-life issues

When my friend Sandy was near the end of her life, I brought her for the second or third time some homemade chicken soup, which she requested. This delighted me because I so earnestly wanted to help and felt honored that my soup was one of the few things she would eat. But once I was seated in her living room across from this beautiful woman lying on a white sofa, which showed off her thick black hair and her signature red lipstick, I was humbled when, after just a few minutes, she said, "Can we not talk? I just need to lie here. I'd like to have you with me, but activity bothers me." I was so grateful to Sandy for being honest with me—she was a straightforward, pull-no-punches fierce, never-smoked lung cancer advocate. But not everyone can be so honest.

As I learned in June 2010 when my father was dying of leukemia, talking with and supporting people in the process of letting go of life can be heart wrenching and tremendously difficult, especially when it is someone you love as much as life itself. This is a subject that deserves much greater attention, as do all of the issues addressed in this section, but it is so much more delicate that I urge you to check the resource section of my website for additional books and articles that may help.

For now, remember the principles woven throughout this book: listen, take your loved one's communicative lead, offer your presence and undivided attention, learn about the dying process (The Hospice Foundation of America provides an excellent, free booklet), and heed this, offered in "Facing Up to the Inevitable, In Search of a Good Death," an outstanding column by Jane Brody in the *New York Times*:

"As someone nears the end of life, it is not unusual to turn inward and become less communicative, even as much as three months before death. Ms. Pitorak [Elizabeth Ford Pitorak, director of the Hospice Institute of Hospice of the Western Reserve in Cleveland] noted that loved ones should not confuse this withdrawal with rejection. Rather, she said, it reflects the dying person's need to leave the outer world behind and focus on inner contemplation." Again, do not take anything personally.

The insights of therapist Halina Irving are of great value as well. "Even people who are dying, you can see they find comfort when they feel understood and when their feelings are being accepted. That relates back to that whole issue of the connection with another person, which is the only thing that gives us solace and comfort.

"I have talked with dying people who have felt so alone because every time they've tried to talk about the fact that they are dying and they want to take care of business—they want to say their final good-byes—their families feel threatened and then say, 'Don't say that, don't talk about it, don't talk negatively,' and they then die isolated and alone."

No one wants to live alone. And certainly no one wants to die alone. Be there.

25.
Cancer in Different Circumstances

In the workplace

A FEW YEARS AGO I WAS asked to consult on a caregiver survey sponsored by AFLAC insurance. The purpose was to determine words and actions that were most and least helpful to unpaid family caregivers. One of the most memorable findings from the nine hundred respondents was that the people caregivers perceived to be least helpful were colleagues and bosses. Not surprising, really, when you consider that your coworkers don't choose to have you in their life. Although some may become good friends, others may become rivals. Most remain casual acquaintances. Because coworkers often bear the brunt of a colleague's illness and subsequent absence, the workplace is understandably the least likely place to find compassion and support.

That said, many who answered my survey found their employers and colleagues tremendously supportive. (When I had cancer, I was self-employed, so did not have to worry about losing my job, but did worry about losing my income. Fortunately, the owners and the human resources director, Alma Azarcon, at Give Something Back Office Supplies made it clear that there would be work waiting for me after my recovery.)

The following comments from my surveys provide gentle and not so gentle guidance for employers and coworkers:

"When I returned to work, my girlfriends there were so protective. They wanted to make sure I wasn't working too hard and that people didn't come up and say dumb things. They were my gatekeepers, so to speak, and they did an effective job."

"I went back to work afterward and most people seemed to ignore what I was going through. I think they were uncomfortable asking, but acknowledging that I was going through some tough times would have been nice."

"The day I returned to the office after my second chemo treatment and wearing my wig for the first time, my boss asked me, 'How many more days do you think you will need to take off? We want to support you, but we have a business to run. . . .' At that moment, I decided that I needed the company for my paycheck and my insurance. I decided that I would look for a new job once I was past my treatment."

"I needed people to let me handle my emotional reaction to the diagnosis the way I wanted to react. At first, for example, I tried to explain to my employer that she needed to get someone in so I could train them to take over my duties. I told her we all needed to hope for the best, but still plan for the worse . . . She didn't want to hear that. She didn't want to hear that I might not survive . . . but at the time I needed her to."

On the phone and online

It's easier for many of us to show compassion and support when we're face-to-face with someone who has cancer. By staying silent, we demonstrate deep caring; indeed, simply laying your hand lightly atop a friend's can be worth many more than a thousand caring words. So what do you do when there really are no words, but you're on the phone and you sort of *have* to say something?

What I often say is something like, "I don't know what to say. I'm so sorry you're going through this and I want to go through it with you. If I were there with you, I'd hold you."

When you're online or messaging with someone, try writing the same thing. Or this evergreen message, written by New Zealand writer Katherine Mansfield nearly a century ago: "This is not a letter [email] but my arms around you for a brief moment."

Better yet, if you're a GD (geographically desirable) friend, offer to come visit, take your friend to lunch or tea, or run an errand for her. Just don't refrain from calling or messaging because you don't know what to say.

And if you get voicemail or decide to email or message your friend, make sure you let her know that you do not demand or expect a response.

Social gatherings

A question I'm often asked is "Is it a good idea to bring up a friend's cancer in a social setting?" If it looks like your friend is having fun, give it a rest. The statement people with cancer most want others to know is "I need to laugh—or just forget about cancer for a while." Let them be the one to bring it up. For further discussion, please refer to chapter 20, "I don't know if I'm cured, and bringing up my health can bring me down," but for now, the following story may provide some insight.

Patricia and Ewan were enjoying a dinner reunion with two old friends, Jackson and Paula. It had been almost two years since Patricia had completed her cancer treatment. "It was one of the first full days that I hadn't given even a thought to the disease that had darkened my soul like chimney soot," she recalled. "Even though the chimney will never be cleaned out completely, I had managed to escape its claustrophobic feel and was thoroughly relishing the light and air on the other side."

Then, just as she was about to dip her spoon into the chocolate pot de crème, it happened: the moment many cancer survivors fear as much as a child fears a shot in her bottom.

"So, Patricia, when do you go to the doctor again?" Jackson asked. It felt like a gut punch. She had finally managed to forget that she would have to return for medical tests every six months for the rest of her life, and suddenly, she found herself smack back in Cancerland.

"I'd rather not talk about that right now," Patricia told him matter-of-factly, instantly losing her appetite. She laughed now as she said, "On the positive side, at least he saved me from consuming those thousand-plus calories!"

Though she wanted to forget about the calamitous disease that had defined her as a victim for almost two years, Patricia could not reclaim the levity or lightness of just one minute before.

Chance meetings

When someone is in the midst of cancer treatment, it can be challenging to know whether to ignore the elephant in the room or bring up a subject that might be terribly upsetting. It can be especially awkward when you run into someone in a public place like a grocery store. But instead of disappearing down the frozen food aisle because you don't know what to say, open your heart, ears, and eyes, and ask casually, "How's it going?" You should be able to tell whether the person wants to discuss his or her health. Does your friend answer tentatively, "Well, I'm okay, I guess," perhaps inviting further questions such as, "Do you want to talk about anything?" If you can't discern a cue, and feel uncomfortable prying (which is rarely a good idea), the best way to proceed is to say with all sincerity something that will tell your friend you genuinely care, such as, "I'm so glad I ran into you. I've been thinking about you."

Money matters

When you have cancer, money fears arise in a major way. Remember, when you're traumatized, you regress emotionally and fear more for your safety. So anything friends and family can do to assuage money fears is tremendously helpful. An experience I had soon after the end of my treatment illustrates this well.

My moods were still mercurial when my husband took me to a spa in Guerneville for my birthday, pampering me all weekend with gourmet meals, a massage, and a hair treatment. The stylist's strong fingers whisking a lather on my scalp soothed me, but when he started pushing pricey hair products, I began to feel pressured, frightened, and put out.

"I just had cancer," I snapped, "so I really have to watch my budget."

"Oh, I am so sorry!" he exclaimed, immediately vanishing behind a curtain to the back room, reappearing a moment later with an outstretched palm proudly holding a cellophane-wrapped gift pack of lemon verbena–scented Pevonia products.

"I have so many friends who have had AIDS and cancer. I know how hard it must be when you can't work and earn money like you used to."

I kept one of the little jars, with just a thumbnail of lotion remaining, because it smelled like love to me.

When you go out for lunch with a friend who has cancer, you can offer to pick up the check, even if you think he's in a higher tax bracket, saying, "You get it next time," clearly implying that there will *be* a next time. Buy a gift, and spend more than you would on yourself. If you have a vacation home, offer it up for free. (When my friend Marcie had cancer, her brother offered her his villa in Tuscany, along with frequent flyer tickets for her and her husband.) You will not be sorry when you see the look of joy and gratitude on your friend or loved one's face!

26.
Cancer at Different Ages

ALTHOUGH IT GOES WITHOUT SAYING that there is no good kind of cancer, and no good age at which to be diagnosed with it, it may feel more tragic, be more painful, and severe, and require different poultices among individuals of different ages. In this section, we consider cancer through the lens of life stages.

Children and cancer

Cancer is cruel, unfair, and odious, no matter whom it strikes, but when it befalls those who should be enjoying the time of life when responsibilities are few and enjoyment is perhaps most pure and authentic, it's almost too much to bear. Children undergoing cancer treatment have to adjust on many levels. Younger children may fear separation from parents during hospitalization. In older children, losing hair or weight may affect their confidence and social stature. Fortunately, children tend to be more resilient than adults, and just as their bodies heal more quickly, so do their spirits.

How do you support the spirit of a child who has cancer? I asked this of Dina Hankin, PhD, Psychologist in Oncology at Children's Hospital and Research Center Oakland, where several hundred children with cancer are treated yearly.

"This is a tricky question and what I recommend is that friends, family, and loved ones ask the parents about what vocabulary they use with their children about their treatment and diagnosis," Dr. Hankin responded. "Particularly when the children are younger, their parents protect them much more. So, for example, parents might not use the word 'cancer' with their children. In this case, close people in the child's life should not . . . use the word with the child. I encourage adults to be open and honest with their child and to use the vocabulary that the child might hear from their doctors, as the child may lose trust in their family and friends if it is not okay to talk about the things they hear in the medical environment. . . . A helpful strategy is for people to ask themselves how best they can be respectful of the child, their situation, and the family.

"Also [helpful is] spending time with children and playing with them. Children going through cancer treatment are often isolated due to infection risk. However, if you have a child that can go play with them, it helps lift their spirits. Showing interest in them about things other than their cancer is helpful, too. Teenagers, in particular, can become tired of only talking about cancer. So, asking about their other interests and helping them to experience other things is helpful. Last, it is all right to have expectations of children going through cancer and to set limits with them. Structure is also important to all children, but particularly when their life is so unpredictable."

In *Armfuls of Time: The Psychological Experience of the Child with a Life-Threatening Illness*, psychologist and associate professor Barbara M. Sourkes, PhD of Lucile Packard Children's Hospital and Stanford Hospital and Clinics helps illuminate, partly through dozens of children's drawings, what it is like for a child to battle cancer. "Drawing is a familiar task for this age group and serves as a powerful means of expression. It often goes beyond the verbal level, enabling the emergence of profound realizations," wrote Dr. Sourkes. This book is highly recommended for anyone wishing for a powerful infusion of compassion and insight.

Parents of children with cancer

Some might say that it's worse to be a care provider for someone with cancer than to be fighting cancer oneself. I've seen it from both sides and could argue either way. What I cannot argue, or even imagine, is what it is like to be a parent of a child who is fighting cancer. To call it a parent's worst nightmare is to minimize a pain that penetrates more deeply than the unconscious mind, cutting to the very core of one's being.

It's not something that any parent of a well child would gladly or even grudgingly imagine, but if you know a parent of a child with cancer, I think it obligatory to do so.

I became acquainted with two women who had children with cancer. Shannon Kelley-Barry wrote a powerful essay, "What Not to Say to the Parent of a Child with Cancer," which she has granted me permission to reprint here. It will be followed by a short piece written by another acquaintance-turned-friend, Mimi Avery. Mimi writes a blog, Julian's World, on CarePages.com. Mimi's commitment to advocate for children with cancer continued and grew after her son, Julian, died, and I asked her if she would write a piece for this book, because I couldn't imagine anyone who could compose anything more heartfelt, honest, and helpful.

Please read both pieces before you even consider talking with a parent whose child has had cancer.

What Not to Say to the Parent of a Child with Cancer
by Shannon Kelley-Barry

My son was diagnosed with brain cancer in April 2006, just a month after his tenth birthday. Even though he was flown from San Antonio to Houston, Texas—to the MD Anderson Cancer Center, no less—it took me a couple of days to get it through my head that my child had cancer. I kept thinking, "It's going to be a benign growth . . . nothing malignant." Seriously, how could my perfectly healthy son have cancer, right?

Wrong. Keeghan's tumor was malignant. But after two surgeries, six weeks of radiation, and a year (so far) of chemotherapy, he is tumor free. It will be my daily—hourly?—wish, for the rest of my life, that he stays that way.

One of the hardest things to deal with when your child has cancer is the way in which other people react when you tell them, and the things that they say. It has been proven to me time after time that most people really don't think before they open their mouths. They'll say things like, "Oh, I knew someone that had the 'C' word. She died."

The "C" word. I've heard cancer referred to that way numerous times, as though actually saying it would cause a person to get it. It's not contagious, people!

At the grocery store one day, with Keeghan standing by my side, the cashier asks me, "Did he have an accident?"

Keeghan has a very large scar on the side of his head. It's a nice scar as far as scars go. It's perfectly symmetrical—four inches up on one side, five inches across, and another four inches down on the other side. It's so perfect that my husband used to joke and say that it looked like a trap door. He'd tease Keeghan by telling people that that was where he kept his wallet.

So to be asked if he had an accident seemed pretty ludicrous. "Yes, he fell out of a tree and landed on a cookie cutter. Hence the perfect scar."

I wish I had replied that way, but alas, I didn't. "He had a brain tumor," I say instead.

"Oh . . . is he going to be okay?" she then whispers.

Keeghan is ten years old. He has cancer. But he's not deaf, nor is he a complete idiot! And he's standing right next to me! Don't talk about him like he's not there or can't understand you. He can. In fact, if you talk directly to him, he can answer any questions you might have about his story quite well. Luckily for me Keeghan replied to the woman's question with a very ten-year-old appropriate, "Yep, I am."

After the first three months of Keeghan's treatment was finished, and before he started his year-long consolidation chemotherapy regimen, we moved from Texas to Washington, DC. Not long after we moved into our house, we got new neighbors. The kids and I were leaving the house to head to the hospital for chemo on the day I met the new neighbor Bob. He noticed that Keeghan had no hair, and that he wasn't looking very happy. Keeghan never looks thrilled when he's heading for chemo. Go figure.

I am of the opinion that it is better to just tell people up front that he has cancer rather than leave them trying to figure out how to ask. So I told Bob, "He has cancer—we're on our way to the hospital now for his chemo treatment so he's not in a very good mood."

Bob asks, "What kind of cancer?" I reply that it is brain cancer.

"Oh, wow. My old boss just died of that."

I can only imagine what the look on my face was. Incredulous, I'm sure. I was so glad that the kids were in the car by that time.

"Are you completely stupid?" is what I should have asked the guy.

"Well, we're hoping that isn't going to happen to Keeghan" was what I actually said. I've come to learn in the few months that we've now been neighbors that Bob never thinks before opening his mouth, so it wasn't just that one incident. But that is the one that sticks in my mind.

Maybe there should be an awareness ribbon for foot-in-mouth disease. What color would it be—flesh? I don't think that color is taken yet. Or perhaps someday I'll write a book and call it "What Not to Say to the Parent of a Child with Cancer." I doubt anyone would buy it though. Everyone thinks they know the right thing to say all the time.

So maybe I should title it, "Hey YOU! Don't Be Stupid!" That might at least get someone to pick it up and read the back cover.

Maybe there's no hope at all and people will continue forever to put their feet in their mouths. But perhaps a little awareness can turn the tide of stupidity.

Lil' King Julian
by Mimi Avery

Nothing could have enraged me more than hearing the words, "He is in a better place, Mimi, you know that right?" at my four-year-old's funeral. What better place is there for a four-year-old than his momma's lap, his daddy's shoulders, or on the playground with his brothers?

He was three years and ten months old when I heard the words, "They found something suspicious in the back of his brain, a mass, the size of a golf ball. We are being admitted."

Those words came from my husband on March 5, 2007, and Julian, our little boy, was about to be diagnosed with brain cancer. Four days later, Julian underwent brain surgery and after eight hours the mass was "totally" removed.

On March 13, we learned a new word: "medulloblastoma," rare and aggressive pediatric brain cancer. I handled the word "mass," I handled the hospital stay, I even handled the surgery, but hearing that my baby had cancer was devastating. Learning that radiation therapy and chemotherapy were in his near future was terrifying.

A four-year-old fighting brain cancer was something I had never heard of and this four-year-old just happened to be my child. It had to be a nightmare, it just couldn't happen to him, to us. . . .

Julian was a trooper, a tough little man. We, as parents, did what we needed to do to make sure he got better and still got to enjoy being a little boy. We watched him lose hair and weight through radiation. We watched the poison dripping into his body. Friends told us over and over that we were strong and that they NEVER could handle it. I would quote to them, "You never know how strong you are, until being strong is the only choice you have." When this happens to you, you do what you have to do. What

I really wanted to say was, "PLEASE stop saying that. I don't want to have to be strong, I want this to all go away!"

Julian was supposed to have a year of treatment; unfortunately, he wasn't even half way through when the beast came back.

"Don't lose hope, it will be all okay. He will be fine," some said. By then I had read every study on relapsed medullo. He wasn't going to be fine and hearing it from people who hadn't been in our shoes didn't help, but as long as Julian was living, I wasn't going to stop fighting for him. But my baby boy was tired: tired of the meds, tired of struggling. His body had had enough. We tried a couple of different oral chemotherapies, with little hope. Eventually, Julian was robbed of all his abilities: walking, using the bathroom, holding his favorite toys and blankies, thinking well, and finally, his life. He was four and died, killed by cancer.

He was my "lil' man," my sunshine, my life.

Three years have gone by without him. Each day is a challenge. Most of my friends are now cancer parents. We often talk about the inappropriate things said to us, hurtful words, stupid words, off-the-wall words, usually said by well-meaning people who believe they HAVE TO talk to make us feel better.

I will share a few of these words with you and maybe when you meet one of us you will remember.

When our children are diagnosed, please don't disappear; we need you then. Come and sit in the hospital with us for an hour. Let us do the talking, we will need to vent.

You might think you can't handle it. Remember, it isn't about you, it is about the children. Find the strength to walk through the hospital doors; we didn't have a choice.

Don't tell us how horrible and difficult it was when your grandmother (or your dog!) had cancer. We understand it might have been, but our children are supposed to grow up and hopefully be old enough to eventually be grandparents.

When our children relapse, we and our doctors look at every possible option to fight again. We spend days and nights looking for the best treatment, so please try to refrain from giving us advice on what we should or should not do.

Reading the words "Stop poisoning your child, let him go" is so painful, just as is being asked, "Why are you stopping treatment, why are you giving up, don't you want to save your kid?" We try our best. The choices, as limited and as difficult as they are, are ours to make. WE have to deal with it for the rest of our lives.

Then, we lose. Our children die. As you stand by their casket, just give us a hug, wipe a tear, no need to talk. As we look at their little bodies, once full of life but now cold and so very still, we don't want you to tell us how beautiful they look. We know what you are trying to say, but there is nothing beautiful about the face of a lifeless child.

They aren't beautiful, they aren't in a better place, and you don't know how we feel if you haven't lost a child. Again, losing your dog doesn't compare.

After the funeral, everyone goes home and eventually back to their lives. Ours stop. Nothing is ever the same and neither are we. The phone calls and visits seem to slow down and eventually stop. I have never experienced it, but a few of my friends, mothers of cancer angels, were told "to move on" and "get back to the living." I can't even understand that someone would think it's okay to say that to a grieving mother.

If we have other children, they keep us going; we don't have a choice but to get up every morning. BUT having other children doesn't lessen the pain of losing one. I don't think I could handle hearing one more time, "At least you have other children," or "Mimi, you still have three boys who need you." I know those facts, I gave birth to the other boys. But whether you have other children or not, when one of your babies die, part of you dies as well. Some of my friends who lost their only child got nauseous as they heard people telling them, "Well, you are still young, you can have more kids."

Instead of trying to fix us, how about listening to us, how about letting us talk about our angels, how about telling us what YOU remember about them. Don't pretend they were never here. . . .

NOTHING and NO ONE can replace our babies.

So please, please, if you ever meet us, remember, watch what you say.

We aren't as strong as you think, we get hurt easily.

Mention our children's name. We might tear up but it's okay, we need to know they aren't forgotten.

Cancer in young adults

Each year, more than seventy thousand people aged fifteen to thirty-nine are diagnosed with cancer and more than ten thousand die of the disease. These grim survival statistics have not changed in the last decade, but just as compelling and unacceptable are the personal, emotional, and lifestyle challenges that young cancer survivors face as they enter the terrifying world sometimes called Cancerland, or as Heidi Adams named it, "Planet Cancer."

Heidi landed there at age twenty-six after enduring excruciating pain in her ankle for eight months before finally being diagnosed with Ewing sarcoma. She would experience a different kind of pain in the coming year.

"My friends were great," Heidi told me. "My brothers are great. But that connection was on a completely different level." No one really understood what she was going through, and although she attended a support group, most of the members could have been her grandparents. She only met four other young adults with cancer throughout her year-plus treatment regimen—two of them while she was undergoing chemo.

It was a few years later, when she was back on terra firma, that she realized she was not as alone as she thought. "I met some folks who were at a foundation with Memorial Sloan-Kettering and who were specifically looking at young adults, and that was the first time the light bulb went off, like 'Oh, yeah, there's probably a lot of people around the country and around the world who went through the same thing I did and we should be able to find each other.'"

In 2001, she helped create a way for young adults with cancer to find each other through a website, Planet Cancer. Young adults could land there and learn more about needs and experiences unique to other people their age. A year later she added a message board, introducing interactivity to the celestial Cancersphere. She said that made it much more than a website: now it was a movement.

In 2003, it claimed a membership of five hundred. Today, it claims upward of five thousand and is more like a universe of diverse nebula where the under-forty set can shop, read, interact, be entertained, laugh, listen, and watch, on demand.

"It allows the element of control," Heidi said. "You can seek what you need when you want it, that 24/7-support on demand. You don't have to wait until 7 o'clock next Tuesday. If you need information, if you need someone to talk to, if you need to get something off your chest, you can just go right then and there in any way you want to. You can use video if that appeals to you, but you know when you feel like shit and you look like shit and you probably don't want to do a video, so video is just another tool that is accessible to young people and it's so helpful."

Other online sites such as The Stupid Cancer Show on Internet radio, which now boasts more than half a million listeners, and organizations such as The LIVESTRONG/Young Adult Alliance, founded by the Lance Armstrong Foundation (Planet Cancer has also become a LIVESTRONG initiative), allow young adults to connect, engage, and advocate. (See the Resource section on my website for more information.) Several books about young adult cancer are now available: Heidi Adams and her brother, Chris Schultz, recently cowrote a guide to navigating young adult cancer. And Kairol Rosenthal, who wrote a short piece about young adult cancer for the first edition of this book, published her own outstanding book in 2009, *Everything Changes: The Insider's Guide to Cancer in Your 20s and 30s*.

Kairol asked me if she could revise what she originally wrote for this book, and I'm thrilled to introduce an improved version of something I thought needed no improvement. For a comprehensive but concise course on how to support a young adult with cancer, read on.

What Young Adults Need You to Know
by Kairol Rosenthal

I recently sat in a café enjoying a juicy hamburger. The restaurant was packed so I ate at the bar. An elegant sixty-something woman sitting next to me struck up a conversation and asked what I did for a living. "I'm an author. I write about young adult cancer," I replied. Everybody knows somebody who has cancer, and she told me about her friends living with this disease. They were patients in their late fifties, sixties, and seventies. Next she added, "It doesn't matter at what age you get cancer. Cancer is cancer. We all have hopes and dreams and when cancer interrupts, age is of no consequence."

I strongly disagree with her. Living with cancer is vastly different at different ages and it is important you understand why. You need to know this information not because one age group deserves more sympathy than another. But because you will be much more successful at helping the young adult cancer patients in your life if you better understand how our lifestyles, diseases, and needs are different.

Three weeks before my own cancer diagnosis at age twenty-seven, I left a low-paying admin job to switch career paths. The day after I received my startling diagnosis, I called to arrange for a second opinion. The nurse refused to schedule my appointment. "You have no health insurance," she told me. My former employer forgot to submit COBRA paperwork that would have extended my health insurance coverage.

I had nineteen malignant tumors in my neck and no insurance. I was single and unemployed. I lived alone in a crumbling three-story walk-up in the Bay Area, my family and long-time friends were sheer across the country. My cancer story isn't glamorous. But it is shockingly typical for young adults.

I fought for and eventually obtained insurance, surgery, and treatment. When I was well enough, I ditched my hospital gown, received a travel grant, and wound my way across the United States recording interviews with other young adult cancer patients. On the frontlines, I learned what young adults commonly experience before, during, and after a cancer diagnosis. I never made the career switch I intended prior to my diagnosis. Instead, I became a writer and went on to have my first book, called *Everything Changes: An Insider's Guide to Cancer in Your 20s and 30s,* published.

Part of what I learned about young adult cancer comes from my own experience of scrounging for insurance, reading voraciously about my disease, and having my heart break wondering if I'd ever find a man to love me in spite of my precarious health. [She did!] The rest of what I learned about young adult cancer comes from researching health-care policy, interviewing medical professionals, and, most important, sitting with a voice recorder listening deeply to scores of other young patients. Here is what we want you to know:

FINANCES AND INSURANCE WHEN
YOU'RE YOUNG WITH CANCER

Young adults tend to feel the financial pinch of cancer the hardest. We experience higher medical debt than any other age group. None of us qualify for Medicare, nor are we eligible for government benefits often available to children. The majority of us are working lower-wage jobs with fewer health insurance and disability benefits. Many of us are still in school or just beginning to pay off student loans. We haven't had enough years to bulk up our bank accounts or pad a rainy day fund.

Most young adult cancer patients need financial and insurance counseling. You can assist us by doing the legwork to find the right people to talk to. Stand by our sides and help us absorb and organize the information we obtain. Help us find and apply for grants and scholarships available to young cancer patients. And, in addition to, or in lieu of, sending get well flowers and stuffed animals, consider giving us gift cards to drug stores, grocery stores, and for gas.

CANCER YOUNG AND SINGLE

Being young and single with cancer can be extremely isolating. The dating scene is doubly daunting when you have this disease. And, it is often lonely being stuck at home, sick, while your friends are out flirting and dating. The practical side of being single can be equally if not more challenging. Without a partner as built-in backup, everything from household chores to attending doctor appointments becomes yours to do solo. For most of us, this is our first experience with major illness. Learning to organize the tendrils of our care is a hefty job to do by ourselves.

Issue us an invitation to vent to you about being single with cancer. If we don't want to talk about it we won't, but we'll probably be glad you asked. Take initiative by organizing our friends to help with household chores and accompanying us to medical appointments so we don't have to always be the one asking. Be sensitive to our need for companionship. Offer for us to come stay at your house for a weekend. Or better yet, keep us company by spending a few nights sleeping on our sofas.

FAMILY PLANNING AND JUGGLING CANCER, BABIES, KIDS, AND TEENS

Young adults are prime childbearing age and our reproductive systems might become jeopardized by surgery or treatment. Our paths toward adoption might also be hindered by having cancer as a strike on our medical records. These circumstances can take extra time, energy, and money to navigate, on top of the emotional and financial resources we are throwing at our disease. Talk to us about these issues so you know best how to be sensitive to our needs. Attending your baby shower might be just the trick to take our mind off chemo, or it might make us want to set the room and all your new baby gifts on fire. Either way, please be understanding.

Some young adults with cancer are already parents to babies, kids, or teenagers. The thought of dying and leaving our growing children behind is a horrific one. Don't shun us for thinking about this. Don't tell us to look on the bright side. Please let us talk about these fears if we need to. On the practical side of parenting with cancer, this illness can cause cabin fever for the whole family. Help by taking our kids for the day to give them a vacation from cancer. Offer to babysit when we have treatment, doctor appointments, or just need an hour at home alone. Or better yet, assemble a babysitting team to cover our regular child-care needs.

CANCER AND YOUNG CAREERS

Cancer patients often hear that this disease can be an awakening, giving new meaning and priorities to life. This notion can be extremely anticlimactic for young adults who are often on our first rungs of the career ladder. Taking time off for our health-care needs can result in missing promotional opportunities or having huge gaps on our resume. After treatment, many of us feel trapped in jobs we may not like but we need in order to maintain health insurance and pay off medical bills. We might need a good sounding board to talk about our fears and frustrations around our bosses, coworkers, and navigating the career world. Don't worry—you don't have to have the answers to our problems, just be a caring listener, and ask us if we'd like your help in locating free legal counseling or free job coaching targeted to cancer patients and employment.

YOUNG BODIES AND YOUNG BIOLOGY

With cancer, it isn't always true that younger patients will do better. Some cancers, such as breast cancer, are actually more aggressive in younger adults than in older adults. Twenty- and thirty-somethings are also frequently diagnosed at later, more aggressive stages of cancer because doctors often don't take our symptoms seriously and delay testing and diagnosis. Young adult cancer research is severely underfunded compared to research for pediatric and older adult patients. As a result, doctors often toss our cases, treatments, and prognoses together with patients who are either decades older or younger than us and whose biology is significantly different than ours.

The solutions to these problems are long-term and systemic. In the meantime, you can help us by not making assumptions about our stamina or prognosis based on our age. Instead, ask open-ended questions about how we are doing and feeling, and read about cancer in young adults from authoritative and reliable medical sources.

YOUNG ADULTS AND SHIFTING SUPPORT SYSTEMS

Young adults move a lot. We are leaving home to go to school, relocating for new jobs, to be with new partners, or just to forge an identity as an adult independent from our parents. If we are not moving, many of our long-time friends are. Our twenties and thirties is also a time when many of us redefine our relationship to spirituality. Some of us are leaving behind the places that as children we called our spiritual homes. It can be really hard to know where our support system is in the midst of such great flux. We have not had decades to build the deep networks of social support held by cancer patients the age of our parents and grandparents.

Help us understand that we can count on you day or night. Give us plenty of examples of the concrete ways in which you can lend a hand. And above all, learn how to listen deeply and without judgment. Not everyone wants a support group. Not everyone wants to talk about their cancer or express their feelings even to friends. But show us that you will be there for us if we want it.

⌐⌐⌐

Women in their childbearing years

As Kairol Rosenthal noted earlier, chemotherapy can damage a woman's reproductive system. Understanding the painful challenges faced by premenopausal women can help you provide loving support. The following essay was written by a dear friend who asked I not share her name. Just so you know, she met the man of her dreams soon after writing this, and married him about a year later.

Cure vs. Kids

When I got the final results of my biopsy for non-Hodgkin's lymphoma, it confirmed I had a more aggressive form than originally indicated, so I was put into chemotherapy a few days later. There were no discussions about harvesting my eggs or doing anything else to preserve my fertility. I was told later there simply wasn't time. At thirty-seven, I was unmarried but still hoping to have children. At the very least, I did not want that possibility taken away from me. My doctors, while kind, were understandably less concerned about my fertility than about getting rid of my cancer. It was difficult for me to hear about the fertility problems of friends because that was the biggest problem in their life. For me, it was simply a side effect of my treatment. I became one of those people who have a problem so big that something like having children would be considered a luxury. I was supposed to be content just to be alive.

My periods stopped sometime around the second course of chemo. I went through the process pretty smoothly, rarely showing any signs of sadness or fear. In the middle of chemo, I went to Stanford University for a second opinion. The doctor commented how well I was responding, but suggested extending the number of rounds because of the large size of my original tumor. I knew that with each successive round, my chances of getting my menstrual cycle back would diminish. But I knew I could not consider that in the decision. She told me that at my age, the chances of remaining in permanent menopause were fifty-fifty. And even if I did get my cycle back, the damage to my eggs and follicles could leave me sterile. After the appointment, I went out to lunch with my parents and burst into tears over a plate of pasta.

My hormone levels put me squarely in menopause. I would joke about my hot flashes with women in their fifties. I saw my gynecologist and a reproductive endocrinologist to discuss hormone replacement therapy. But about a month or so later, I started feeling a familiar sensation I usually got at the onset of my period. The day it began, I had not been as excited as I was since I was fourteen and a half and was convinced I was the last girl in high school to menstruate. After getting monthly periods for about nine months, I returned to my gynecologist for some additional tests. I found out that not only had my hormone levels returned to normal, but that there was every indication that I was ovulating. Once again, I burst into tears.

I do not know if I will have children, or at least bear them considering I am near the end of my biological clock. I am even considering the possibility of having them on my own. But my point is that I feel blessed that I still may have a choice—that cancer has not taken this away from me. While nobody said this with anything other than good intentions, I get the sense from other people that they feel I should not worry about this and just be grateful to be alive. I am grateful. But I think the reason that I get so upset is that it hits me on a deep level, as a cancer survivor and as a woman. I let my emotions go about my fertility and hormonal problems in a way I can't about the cancer.

Cancer in the Golden Years and beyond

Cancer is heinous and harrowing no matter how old you are. But as tough as it is, many seniors are quick to acknowledge their good fortune to have lived as long as they have. "I've had eighty-three years," said my father, after learning he would soon die of acute myeloid leukemia. "A lot of people don't get that. I've had a great life."

Even so, most of us cringe when we hear any sentence prefaced with "At least . . ." as in "At least he had a good life," "At least he doesn't have young children," or "At least he's leaving a legacy of a wonderful family." Although such statements may be intended to point us toward the bright side, they more often come across as diminishing the magnitude of an imminent, massive, and incomprehensible loss.

It doesn't bother me when people ask how old my father was when he died—and that's usually the first question people ask, as if they need to know where to place him on the tragedy timeline—but I still can't help but think that, no matter when someone dies, it's almost always too soon.

Yes, Dad had a wonderful life. Yes, he's no longer in pain. Yes, there may be other silver linings hidden behind thick dark clouds. But my father loved life, and whether someone's three or eight-three, cancer sucks. No one should die of it. I guess if there could be a hierarchy of cancer, we'd want to save the women and young people first to ensure our species' survival. But cancer is not a contest. And please don't assume that just because someone is old, they are ready to give up on life. And don't give up hope for them, or abandon them.

Diane Blum, MSW, and Richard Hara of CancerCare reported in a 2009 article, "Social Well Being and Cancer Survivorship" in *Oncology Nurse Magazine*, that 61 percent of cancer survivors are over age sixty-five, but that the research about older adult issues "has not been commensurate with their statistical importance." They attribute this partly to ageism, but also point to complications arising from the fact that symptoms of recurrence or late effects of treatment may be obscured by other health conditions. In addition, they report, "Another practical issue that looms large for older survivors is lack of social support. Many are isolated, socially because they have outlived their significant others and peers, and geographically, either because their family and friends live far away, or they do not have the transportation resources to stay in regular contact with them. When there are family members who could help, they are often encumbered by their own home responsibilities . . . and/or their own health issues (in the case of the spouse/partner of the same age cohort). Transportation to follow-up treatment can thus pose a significant logistic and financial burden on those who have lost their physical and/or financial independence."

Keep this in mind when you hear of a senior neighbor or acquaintance with cancer. Reach out. Be there.

27.
She Wants/He Wants:
Cancer and Gender

IN 1991, I PRODUCED A DOCUMENTARY about the impact of divorce on children. The teenage daughter of a bitter parental parting made more hellish by my mother's chronic depression and her psychiatrist's lack of competent care, I had a personal stake in discovering and sharing what divorcing parents can do to spare their children trauma and, often, decades of psychotherapy.

After completing *Broken Homes, Healing Hearts* and sharing numerous hopeful stories demonstrating that amicable divorces can be had without inflicting deep wounds or lifelong scars, I still remained convinced that it is every parent's responsibility to do everything possible to avoid divorce in the first place (except in the case of abuse). So the aim of my next documentary, *Loving for Life*, was to show how to build and maintain strong marriages.

One of the experts we interviewed was sociolinguist Deborah Tannen, PhD, author of the now classic *You Just Don't Understand: Women and Men in Conversation*, which had just been published. I'll never forget reading her book—I was sitting by a stream bank in a thick redwood forest near the Oregon Coast and was so excited that I couldn't pull myself away from her words, even as the day drew dark and I faced a ninety-mile drive back to Portland. Tannen was instilling hope in me that, a decade after my own divorce, I might still be able to create a love that could last.

Tannen's book traces men and women's differences in conversational style and approach back to childhood, illustrating and explaining how we communicate differently from the time we are toddlers. Without blaming or crediting either sex, but simply exploring differences and endeavoring to facilitate understanding and more effective and satisfying cross-gender communication, *You Just Don't Understand* posits that men and women really can live together in peace and harmony, *if they just understand and respect one another's differences.* To quote Tannen: "Saying that men talk about baseball in order to avoid talking about their feelings is the same as saying that women talk about their feelings in order to avoid talking about baseball."

The book's lessons have remained in the back of my mind since I first read it in 1991; even now, when my husband, David, refuses to ask for directions as we wind through unfamiliar streets in search of an elusive destination, I remember that it is the "one down" position it would put him in, not his stubbornness, that keeps him from stopping. (Thank goodness for GPS, which largely solves the problem in many populated areas.)

I took Tannen's lessons for granted when I wrote the first edition of this book. Although I gave gender a brief nod, I came to believe later that it deserved much more attention. This was reinforced last summer, as I lived through my father's cancer diagnosis and battle and found myself sorely challenged to respect his needs, which were so different from mine when I had cancer.

In digging more, I discovered that new biological science and clinical research supported Tannen's sociolinguistic theories. As I began writing this section, I searched for professionals in cancer care who had addressed gender differences in research and clinical practice who could answer the simple question, "Do men and women with cancer need and want different things?"

Such a simple question. The tendency is to generalize and turn to the work of Tannen and others, which present men as protectors and women as nurturers; men as status and rank-seekers and women as equity, community, and consensus-builders; men as natural advisers and women as sometimes unwilling vessels of male counsel and information. But it's much more complex that that, said Matthew Loscalzo, LCSW, director of an integrated cancer support program at the City of Hope, who has been working in cancer pain management, palliative care, and counseling for thirty years, and who coauthored a book with Marc Heyison, president of Men Against Breast Cancer, *For the Women We Love: A Breast Cancer Action Plan and Caregiver's Guide for Men.* This clear, mission-based book is designed to help men do what they want more than anything else: to help and protect their women.

"It's a complex picture, but it's a magical picture," enthused Loscalzo when we spoke on the phone. "And for people who don't like complexity, it's painful; but for the rest of us who thrive on it, it's a magnificent story. Women and men are great together. They just have to get their expectations more realistic and they both have to be more flexible."

I discovered Loscalzo while searching the Internet for articles about gender and cancer, and found, among the few listings, a 1999 article, "In Coping with Cancer, Gender Matters," from the *Journal of the National Cancer Institute*.

Gender-related ways of coping have "profound differences with important implications in how you engage women and men in the disease process," said Loscalzo in the article, adding that we know almost nothing about how men and women cope. "The whole psychosocial area is virtually ignored . . . we need to understand how women and men integrate stress and cope with it, and we need to learn how they interact and how we can help them do so more effectively."

In the decade-plus since that article came out, Loscalzo's wish has certainly been granted. Not only did the Institute of Medicine recommend in 2008 that all cancer care should include treatment for emotional and social problems caused by the disease, but also research on the brain itself now demonstrates how hormonal and structural differences point to and explain our distinctively different gender-related needs.

There's now a specific field of medicine called "gender-based medicine," and the advent of functional MRI (fMRI) has revolutionized the field. "When you talk and I talk," said Loscalzo, "about three parts of my brain light up, mostly in the left side. When women talk, about eight or nine parts of your brain light up. That's why when women start talking about one thing, they can talk about the next thing, the next thing, the next thing." Men tend to get lost, said Loscalzo, and grow frustrated that women can't stay focused and follow through on one thought.

The fMRI demonstrates other differences. Women verbally process their emotional experience as it happens, while men do not. Men can only process their emotional experience retrospectively. And women are more sensitive to feelings. "Women tend to be able to walk into a room and to pick up the emotional feel of the room rapidly," said Loscalzo. "Men have a much harder time and they miss the obvious things.

"These differences begin before birth, in the hormones that bathe our brains as we develop, he explained. "If we took the chemicals in a male brain and injected them into a woman's, she'd feel very much like a man. If we took the biochemical milieu in a woman's brain and injected it into a man, he'd feel very feminine. And we know this because when we put men on different hormonal therapies, they get hot flashes, they get emotional."

But although we are essentially wired at birth—"You can take a boy in any country and give him a Barbie doll and he's going to bend the legs and make it into a spear or a gun," remarked Loscalzo—we can't really talk about gender in a static way because, like Barbie's legs, we are plastic creatures as well. "Society takes what we are built with and bends it and twists it and teaches us how to react in certain ways. So if you have that young man who is a very sensitive young man, who would cry at the drop of a hat, or that woman who wants to play with boys, society can beat up on them and make them very conflicted beings. So when we think about women and men, we have to think about them on a continuum."

"So how does this translate into action, especially regarding cancer?" a man in particular, might ask, being typically more solution-oriented. Loscalzo answered by referring to his three decades of experience dealing with cancer and gender and running cancer support groups. The men and women meet separately, and then together with their husbands and wives; some are survivors, others are caregivers.

The women might express among themselves anger that their husbands are making jokes about cancer. (A comment from my survey is a perfect example of this: "Right after my mastectomy, when they took off the bandages, my husband looked at the scars and said, 'Oh, look, the Bride of Frankenstein.' I was totally devastated and if there weren't a nurse in the room and I wasn't strung up with drains, I think I would have jumped out of the bed and strangled him. After telling him how insensitive that remark was, he said it was meant to be funny. I thought it was grounds for divorce!")

When the men reenter the room, here's what Loscalzo says to them: "The women really do not like when you make jokes when they're feeling stressed out." He asks the men to explain to the women why they make jokes and use humor the way that they do. Then he asks the women to explain why they try to get their husbands to share how they are feeling, and how it makes them feel when their men protect them by keeping their feelings to themselves.

"And then we say, 'Now women, we need for you to teach the men how it makes you feel when they're protecting you like that.' And the women say, 'It terrifies us. We feel alone, we feel isolated, we feel abandoned, we feel trivialized: it doesn't help us.' And the men are shocked. And the women are shocked when the men say that. Because they just take it so personally. They feel that they're being rejected and not loved and all of a sudden, we have a grownup conversation."

Loscalzo calls this kind of connection—he doesn't call it communication because he thinks it's more about connection—"gender synergy," and explains that it's about getting women and men to get the best out of each other.

"When you have cancer, as you know, the volume is turned up on everything, but also people are more open, changed. They are more open to hearing that the life is fleeting, it's valuable, make every moment count. So we can say, 'Guys, you know, when you left the room we were speaking with the women, and when you guys were in the other room, you were speaking with the men and this is what we came up with.'"

Loscalzo said the best thing for women to do, according to what the men have told him again and again, is to just say, "I love you. I care about you. I want to be helpful. But I'm not going to pressure you. Just know that I'm here and if you want to talk about anything, I want to talk about it, too, but I'm not going to harass you."

"Give men the space and give them the support at the same time," said Loscalzo.

He explained that if women want men to talk, they need to know this: that men avoid anything that they don't have control over, and that they are much more comfortable with feeling angry than feeling sad or feeling hurt, and that if you make them feel vulnerable, they will shut down, unless they have been to therapy or are very open men. (He also said those were generalizations, not stereotypes, but that we at least consider them seriously.)

Loscalzo said men are more likely to allow women to help them if they don't feel they're exposing themselves, but are helping someone else. "So if you want to know how they are feeling, ask them how they think other men would be feeling in that situation. Say, 'We need for you to help us to help other men and to help the women who are helping these men. Can you please give us your guidance and your input?'

"They're coming from a position of strength. For women, a position of vulnerability is not a problem because she sees it as working it out with so many other people, but if you're a man, you're supposed to work this out by yourself. And all of a sudden, that's pretty vulnerable."

Whatever you do, advised Loscalzo, don't tell men how they're feeling, how they should be feeling, or what they should do. "Women have got to realize that whenever a man hears a woman telling him what to do, no matter how what age that woman is—if she's fifteen years younger than him or twenty years older or the same age, she is his mother. So when women suggest and correct men like they do fairly frequently, it's dangerous because the more that person corrects, and becomes like that person's mother, the less that man is going to want to connect with her and emotionally support her and the less he's going to want to have sex with her because now she's become his mother.

Men need to realize that women need different things, too. "If a woman wants to sit and talk, you sit and talk, and if you don't get anything out of it, that's too bad. She's getting something. And if you're a man who has courage, don't tell me running into a burning building means having a lot of courage. It does. But I think more courage is if you really love this person and respect this person, you'll shut up and you'll listen.

Note to men everywhere: Don't try to fix women's problems! We just want to feel heard and cared for. And we want to see that you care. As one woman who answered my survey wrote, "My husband felt he had to be 'the man' and not get emotional with me. I needed him to cry with me and to understand how afraid I was—and let me have that feeling. Ultimately, I had to understand that it was probably too much for him, especially after losing his father so soon before my own diagnosis."

And women, listen to Loscalzo's advice: "What I tell people is whenever you have a woman and a man in a room, you have to say there's a third object in the room and it's the problem we're working on to get together, or else it becomes the woman being the victimized person where they're beating up on her or the guy gets beat up. No, we are a team." Men like teams. And they like to solve problems.

Loscalzo said mutual respect is the ultimate goal. Neither men nor women should judge what the other gender does or how it thinks or operates. It seems so simple, and although it's what I practiced professionally as a documentary producer and journalist—listening without judging—it's far more difficult in relationships, because our emotions and egos are at stake.

Loscalzo got into gender work through his practice in pain management. He noticed that his abstract, feeling-based therapeutic style wasn't working with men—they didn't return for treatment, as his women patients did. "So I changed my therapeutic style to being much more problem solving, not focusing on abstracts, focusing on outcomes, and lo and behold, my caseload totally changed." Then he realized that his success belied a sad failure. "If you think about how many nurses are female—almost all of them—how many social workers are female—almost all of them. How many psychologists are female—almost all of them. And if you look at medical schools, 56 to 60 percent of them are now female and they're expecting to be more, and more, and more, so we have a health system where men are going to feel more alienated, so we don't have enough and men are underserved in terms of their psychological and spiritual needs because we don't understand them."

That is one of the challenges Loscalzo said we face in coming years. In spite of the fact that psychosocial issues are gaining attention, gender differences must be addressed. In 2005, a study was published in *Urologia Internationalis* concerning psychological assessment and gender differences in people with genito-urinary cancers. And more studies are appearing that show men may typically do well by using denial as a defense and may not want to discuss their feelings about diagnosis and treatment, while women need to communicate their thoughts and feelings. But more studies, and more discussion of gender differences in treating and coping with psychosocial issues in cancer care, are sorely needed. In the meantime, read this section again the next time you're going to talk with someone of the opposite sex who has cancer.

A "breast cancer husband's" point of view

Although reading stories about men and women in conversation, and hearing from authorities on gender and cancer inform and enlighten, there's nothing like hearing it from the horse's mouth. Journalist Marc Silver became an authority while researching and after authoring *Breast Cancer Husband*, a book based on his personal experience with the disease. He wrote the following for us, but especially for men.

Cancer Husbands: What You Need to Know
by Marc Silver

I didn't know what to call myself when my wife was diagnosed with breast cancer. She was the patient, the fighter, and ultimately, the survivor.

But who was I? How did my identity change? I stuck a label on myself: "Breast Cancer Husband." That sounded about right. But I had no clue as to what the job entailed.

I thought I should be a cheerleader. You know: Look on the bright side, honey, at least you're only stage 2!

I thought I should be her protector. I should find the best docs and the perfect treatment for her cancer.

I thought I should fix things.

What I found out after my wife was diagnosed with breast cancer is that I couldn't fix anything, I shouldn't make decisions for her, and I definitely got in trouble when I tried to cheer her up. Sometimes, all she wanted to do was tell me how much cancer sucked. And all I needed to say was, "Yup, it sure does."

My wife went through the Big Three treatments: surgery (a lumpectomy in each breast), chemotherapy, and radiation. Today, she is in good health. But back in those dark days, when it seemed that cancer was in charge of our lives, I remember how lost and confused I felt. I didn't know what I was supposed to do. That's why I wrote a book—*Breast Cancer Husband: How to Help Your Wife (and Yourself) Through Diagnosis, Treatment, and Beyond*. It's for all the clueless guys like me, who want to be there when the woman they love is diagnosed with breast cancer but don't know exactly what to do.

Guys, here are some of the lessons I learned.

1. **Shut up and listen.** I call this the breast cancer husband's motto. (Actually, it works well for any husband.) Your job isn't to call the shots. It's to be your wife's support, to tell her what you think when she asks . . . but then understand if she doesn't follow your advice.

2. **Be her appointment pal.** Sitting with your wife in the doctor's office sounds like no big deal, but it turns out to be a Very Big Deal. You are there for her. I came across a study that said that holding your spouse's hand in a stressful situation can help reduce her stress (and maybe yours, too). What's more, you can take notes or tape-record the doctor's visit, so if she doesn't keep all the information in her head—which is perfectly normal for anyone with a critical disease—you can go to the tape. And while you shouldn't ask questions for her, you can keep a list of her questions on hand so you can remind her, as the clock is ticking, of queries she wanted to pose to the doc.

3. **Don't be afraid to come on to her.** Sure, sex isn't always possible during cancer treatment. But it's not impossible, either. If you're in the mood, and she is, for a few minutes you won't be thinking about cancer. And if she's not in the mood, well, as my wife puts it, "Too bad for you." But seriously folks, remember: Cuddling can be a wonderful way to stay physically connected during the months of treatment.

4. **Remember, it ain't over when the last treatment ends.** Lots of men think that the end of active treatment means that cancer is done, gone, kaput. Unfortunately, this is a disease that leaves a psychological imprint. Your wife may be physically exhausted after treatment. She may miss the regular attention of her doctors. And she may be afraid of recurrence. You can tell her, as our oncologist told us, that worrying about recurrence doesn't get you anywhere. If there's no recurrence, you've wasted all that time worrying. And even if there is a recurrence, you've still spent time worrying that you could have spent enjoying life.

28.
Cancer and Cultural Background

A RECENT STUDY OF LATINO MEN showed that their beliefs about masculinity may discourage them from getting screened for prostate cancer. Researchers at the University of Illinois reported, "Complex cultural and gender beliefs about manliness and sexuality that . . . stigmatize the digital rectal exam as emasculating . . . could explain why some men don't seek care until the cancer has progressed, diminishing their chances for recovery." And an article in *The South Florida Sentinel* indicated that Hispanic women may have a higher incidence of cervical cancer than any other group because of sexual mores. Ysabel Duron, who founded Latinas Contra Cancer in California, said this may be due to the taboo about having conversations concerning sex, and that some husbands may prevent their wives from being screened.

Clearly, cultural background does influence how cancer may be perceived, prevented, and treated. But in spite of egregious disparities in survival and access to cancer care among different ethnic groups, the experience and psychosocial needs of people with cancer share some common themes. Goldie Eder, LICSW, a therapist and lecturer in psychiatry at Harvard Medical School, coleads a support group that has included patients from Nepal, one of whom is a former Buddhist monk; a woman from the Philippines, a Brazilian nurse, an African American man in substance abuse recovery, a former milliner and pastry chef, a man from Central America, and a professional with bipolar disorder.

As different as they are, Eder said that what survivors want regardless of cultural background is "reassurance that people have not forgotten that they are still dealing with a life-threatening illness, even after the acute treatment phase of their illness . . . They talk a lot about balancing their needs to focus on their own health versus nurturing/taking care of others. . . . I would describe a lot of the discussion as dealing with the increased sense of uncertainty and ambiguity that dealing with cancer has introduced . . . and the anxiety that can bring."

Nevertheless, in certain cultures, cancer may carry a greater stigma and may still be viewed as a form of punishment or even contagious. And as you will see in the following stories, some people feel that their cultural or ethnic background holds them to behavioral standards that are difficult to meet, and face rejection and loneliness because of superstition and lack of education in their communities.

You have to stay silent

Virginia Mei sifted through more than a half century of memories to recall the day in her homeland of China that the Red Guard came to her door demanding her Bible.

"I was frightened. Had to let them in, give our Bible." The eighteen-year-old had stepped aside to let the three young men climb the narrow stairway to her family's second-floor apartment. "The word of Mao was the word of God," she recalled.

"I was a medical doctor in China," she continued. "I have my college education in the 1950s and 60s in mainland China." Dr. Mei left the party and China after practicing medicine there for fifteen years. She came to the United States to help support her son, who attended college at the University of California at Berkeley, and so that she could freely worship the God she still loved. Her husband would follow as soon as he could get a visa.

Dr. Mei's cousin, a publisher of a local bilingual Chinese American newspaper in San Francisco, hired her as an editor. Although she knew little English, she learned on the job, working extra hours to help pay for her son's tuition.

"I'm so busy that I don't feel that I'm sick. But in my bowels, there was a little bit of fresh blood." She thought she might have hemorrhoids, but deep down in her heart, because she was a doctor, she suspected that it was more serious than that. She lived with her fear for too long, she said. By the time she sought medical attention, the tumor had grown to four and one half centimeters.

"I have to blame myself because I did not go to the doctor," she said angrily. She also felt lonely. "It was all kept inside. Because I was living with my son. He was so busy studying, so I don't want to bother him." The only people she told were her husband, in China, and her pastor and his wife, in San Francisco.

The stigma of cancer, pervasive in her culture, oppressed her. She said it was like living under Communist rule. "Especially in Chinatown, there are some people, they're not well-educated, so they don't understand about cancer. Some people think that it is bad luck, it is contagious. So people just keep the distance. And also, some people just feel that, 'Oh, maybe you've done something very bad and then you got punished.'"

As an educated woman and physician, Dr. Mei neither blamed herself for getting cancer nor thought she was contagious. But the knowledge that she had as a doctor, made her fear something else. "My life expectancy was very low. I wondered, how long can I live?"

Dr. Mei lived and thrived. She became a community counselor and, speaking three different dialects of Chinese—Cantonese, Mandarin, and Shanghai—she enlarged her client base, counseling men, women, and youth from her homeland with family or marriage problems. Then, a few years later, she read a column in the Chinese newspaper written by a woman who got breast cancer and underwent surgery, radiation, and chemotherapy alone, and Dr. Mei wondered, How come we Chinese people don't help each other? That inspired her to create an ongoing cancer support group for Chinese American women to help reduce the stigma of cancer and increase the sense of community so vital to good mental health.

"We want to educate our people that this is just like high blood pressure or diabetes. Everyone has a chance to survive. This is no punishment. We like to have people walking with us through this difficulty. Come walk beside me!"

A thirty-year-old Asian American medical doctor, Lisa, wrote to me after reading about Dr. Mei in the first edition of this book. Almost six months after being diagnosed, Lisa still had not told her own parents about her diagnosis of thyroid cancer. "I'm not sure if or when I ever will. . . . Just wondering if you are still in touch with Virginia Mei, or if she or you know of any other Asian American woman cancer support groups around the country?" I asked her to tell me more about her situation, and she wrote,

"My parents have always been overly protective to a fault. . . . And the health thing is even worse. Neither of my parents go to doctors themselves (though I have diagnosed my dad with gout, hypertension, and shingles over the phone). My mom thinks a cold or a cavity is a huge deal when it happens to any of us children of hers. So I can only imagine what she'll think if/when she finds out I actually had cancer."

This points to why it's imperative that all of us fight the stigma and promote a better understanding of cancer.

You have to lose your hair

Johanna had just earned her master's degree in public policy when her boyfriend, Martin, proposed to her on vacation in Hawaii. They set a wedding date almost a year in advance to make sure their nuptials fit their dreams. Soon after that, Johanna felt a lump in her neck. She said she didn't think it was anything serious, but went to the doctor anyway. He told her not to worry—that it was probably a swollen gland—but a month later, she felt another lump and returned to the doctor, who ordered a biopsy.

"We got the results, and he said I had stage 3 Hodgkin's disease and that I would have to do twelve weeks of chemo and four weeks of radiation," said Johanna. Her shock and sadness deepened into bitter disappointment as she realized she would finish her twelve-week round of chemo on her scheduled wedding day.

"A couple of days after my diagnosis, Martin said, 'What are we going to do, wait until July?'"

Johanna and Martin decided to marry the week before her chemo. That gave them two weeks to prepare. "So we planned a wedding," Johanna laughed. "We had seventy people show up. And the thing that was amazing was that so many people came and helped us with things. Martin's aunt bought my dress. A florist gave us a discount, because she was moved by what was going on. My employer even let us use my building for the reception."

Nine days after her beautiful wedding, she started chemotherapy. "That day, I cut all my hair off, just so when it fell out, I wouldn't have to have it bald long."

Johanna had hair that turned heads a half a block away. Long, black, and curly, it was the result of a gorgeous blend of cultures, an Italian mother and African American father. Her shiny curls grew past her slender waist. Losing what she always considered her most beautiful physical gift and a central part of her identity—her hair—terrified her almost more than anything else she faced. Her well-meaning friends didn't make it any easier.

"I think within the African American community there's especially, for women, a big emphasis on our hair. So when I found out that I had cancer, that was the thing a lot of black women I knew related to. The first thing they would say was, 'Oooooo, you're going to lose your hair? But you have such good hair!' or "Oh, that's horrible!'" Others trivialized her imminent loss by asking, "Why are you being so vain? Why do you even care about this?"

What made it so frightening to Johanna was not only that her hair would fall out, but that it was something totally out of her control. "The doctor said, 'You might become infertile, you might have problems with this or that. But you're definitely going to lose your hair.' I could have hope about everything else, but I knew I was definitely going to lose my hair."

Johanna knew Martin adored her hair, and because he couldn't bear to watch it sheared off, dropped her off at the salon. But the words he spoke upon seeing her assuaged her fear that he would no longer find her attractive.

"'Oh, my God, you're so much prettier! I love it!' he told me. He was so sweet!"

Johanna said the cancer that fueled her fear helped her overcome other fears. "I never would have gone back to get my PhD," she said thoughtfully. "There's never been a black person in the public policy doctoral program, and there have only been thirty-three PhDs in that program ever. I think I would have been way too scared, but now I'm not. I can do chemo. And radiation was in some ways worse than the chemo. So I can do a PhD!"

29.

Other Situations, Complications, and Conditions

Cancer and the soul

MY FAITH IN GOD, or "The Mystery," as I sometimes call it/her/him, strengthened during my bout with cancer. Faith is not something you can impart to a loved one, and many feel betrayed by God when they or someone they love receives a cancer diagnosis. But spirituality of any kind—a walk in the forest, meditation, or other forms of self-care—can be tremendously helpful. The following comments from cancer survivors may give you some ideas about how to support your loved one's spirituality:

"I am a Christian and my faith sustained me through the entire process. I found great comfort that I was not alone even when I was physically alone with my inner thoughts. I also believe that many prayers were said for me and there is power in prayer."

"I wanted reassurance that I would move past this and live a long, happy, healthy life. I wanted to be reassured that despite this bad bump in the road, God would walk me through this. I wanted unconditional love and understanding about what I was going through."

"A friend called with some scripture, which I held onto like a lifeline: Jeremiah, *NIV* Version: *'For I know the plans I have for you, declares the Lord; plans to prosper you and not to harm you; plans to give you hope and a future.'* I also had an abundance of Christian friends, praying for me. They sent me cards and notes, which I kept up on the kitchen counters and that overflowed into the dining room area. I kept these up all through radiation treatments, as a visual reminder that all these people were upholding me in prayer."

"My friend sent me Bible verses and expounded on them to make them apply to me personally. They took me from day one, when I received my diagnosis up through surgery and chemo, and were so comforting and I got such strength from them. I told her afterward that she had held the 'Christ-light' for me through the darkness."

Depression

Cancer treatment may change the way an individual's brain works, actually causing depression. According to the National Institute of Mental Health (NIMH), studies indicate that about 25 percent of people with cancer experience depression, yet only 2 percent of cancer patients in one study were receiving antidepressant medication. "Despite the enormous advances in brain research in the past twenty years," reports a NIMH fact sheet on depression and cancer, "depression often goes undiagnosed and untreated."

The paper continues, "Persons with cancer, their families and friends, and even their physicians and oncologists may misinterpret depression's warning signs, mistaking them for inevitable accompaniments to cancer. Symptoms of depression may overlap with those of cancer and other physical illnesses."

The NIMH says treatment for depression cannot only help people feel better and cope more effectively with the cancer treatment process, but also "there is evidence that the lifting of a depressed mood can help enhance survival. Support groups, as well as medication and/or psychotherapy for depression, can contribute to this effect." (For those who shy away from support groups or who are too ill to attend, there are numerous online support groups that may be helpful. See the Resources section on my website.)

According to a 2009 article in *Science Daily*, graduate student Jillian Satin, MA, at the University of British Columbia in Vancouver, Canada, and her colleagues analyzed all of the studies to date they could identify related to cancer and depression. They found twenty-six studies with more than nine thousand cancer patients that examined the effects of depression on their survival. "We found an increased risk of death in patients who report more depressive symptoms than others and also in patients who have been diagnosed with a depressive disorder compared to patients who have not," said Satin. In the combined studies, the death rates were up to 25 percent higher in patients experiencing depressive symptoms and 39 percent higher in patients diagnosed with major or minor depression.

Stanford Medical Center psychiatrist and researcher David Spiegel, MD told me about a recent study he completed that was published in the *Journal of Clinical Oncology*. It looked at changes in depression in cancer patients, measuring the chronicity and severity of the depression. "Basically, if you use the pattern of depression getting better or staying the same in that year, you could significantly predict mortality up to ten years later independent of all the other risk factors, independent age of diagnosis—and so on. Depression independently predicted mortality."

Lawrence LeShan, PhD, divides depression into two types, realistic and neurotic, and said they can overlap. "Most cancer depression is realistic. Most people who get cancer were raised when getting cancer was an absolute disaster. With neurotic and psychological depression, the best thing is antidepressants. With realistic depression, you may occasionally use antidepressants as a start-up point, a jump start. You say, 'Alright, let's get some action, let's do this.'

Dr. LeShan said antidepressants are very useful to "jump-start" treatment, but depressive illness cannot be changed by medications. "They make the immune system function better because you feel better, because they mask the depression. That masking is marvelous, because then you start acting in such a way that you find more enthusiasm in your life."

If a cancer patient resists taking medications, Dr. LeShan suggests saying something like the following to your friend or loved one: "You seem depressed; you don't feel like moving. It's not good for you. You may not feel like you care that much right now, but if there's something you would like to do if you weren't depressed, I'll go to with you the first time. If it's too much trouble to get your car out of the garage, I'll take it out for you the first time, then I'll get the hell out of your way."

Again, most important is that you be there for your loved one. Few people want to be told what to do, but gentle suggestions made with love, after asking permission to make such suggestions, may be deeply appreciated. (See Dr. Wendy Harpham's advice in chapter 9.)

Also vital is that you recognize and accept that depression is to be expected. Said one woman who responded to my survey, "I would have liked to have heard that it was normal to have feelings of depression."

Parents with cancer

When I was diagnosed with cancer, The Cancer League, a volunteer organization of women impacted by cancer, donated a grant in my honor to East Bay Agency for Children and the Women's Cancer Resource Center to support a program to help teens whose parents have had cancer. I was deeply touched, heartened, and grateful, not only because my son would be able to attend the group, but because other youth would benefit from the support. I knew that, although the tendency among friends and loved ones of people with cancer is to offer support to the person who actually has the disease, most survivors who have children know their sons and daughters need help just as much. You can help your loved one by searching out programs that support children and teens online as well as face-to-face, and the following comments from my survey respondents point out practical ways to offer support:

"I wanted parents of my kids' friends to perhaps offer to do the driving to sports and offer to pick up the practice schedules at parent meetings and that sort of thing."

"Food was helpful for my family . . . but not always casseroles, which most children don't eat. My kids could have used more distractions. People should have been inviting them to the movies and fun activities just to get them out of the house."

"Helpful were the friends and family who provided babysitting for my two-year-old, food and house cleaning and support for my husband."

"I appreciated people who offered to help get my kids, who were quite young then, from place to place."

For doctors and health-care providers only

One could certainly write an entire book about how medical professionals can best relate to, support, and communicate with cancer patients—and indeed, several books have been written by physicians, including Christina

Puchalski and Wendy Harpham—but the following comments collected from my survey and other sources, speak volumes.

"After my mastectomy, my surgeon came in and the first words out of his mouth were, 'Good Morning, Beautiful.' It comforted me so to think that I might be beautiful even though at that moment I felt mutilated."

"There was a guy who tattooed me for the radiation who said he couldn't understand why people minded it. And then his hand slipped and the mark is bigger than need be. I thought he was a fool not to realize why we'd mind—a permanent reminder of a very scary time."

"When I was first diagnosed, the nurses were in the recovery room with me. My stupid surgeon with the compassion of a gnat lifted the oxygen mask off my face and said, 'yeah, it was cancer but we got it all,' and walked off. I started crying, it was the amazing and compassionate nurses who came over to me and comforted me with their own survivor stories of this illness. Thank GOD for them! They lifted my spirits and gave me hope."

"I liked it if the personnel doing the surgery or radiation were kind and reassuring but didn't treat me like an overly anxious person. I remember an operating room nurse who spoke to me before the final surgery and was so reassuring just telling me her name, what would happen, that I would be able to ask questions until I went under, and then, when they were doing all the things they do on the table, she kept checking in with me."

"About a month before [my dad] died, he saw one of the doctors at the clinic. [The doctor] had the audacity to tell my dad and my mom that if he 'just had a better attitude and tried a little harder, he would get better.' What you don't know is that my dad was one of the most positive people I had ever known in my life. Yes, he shed many tears of sorrow, but he never forgot about all of the blessings that God had given him in his sixty-two years of life. He fought a really hard battle for twenty-six months, he never wanted to give up—but eventually it beat his body—not his spirit!"

"In preparation for radiation, they do a CT scan of the chest area. Three weeks after that, I was meeting with the radiologist and he says, 'Oh, by the way, you have some spots on your liver that we saw on the CT scan.' I knew that [breast cancer] metastasizes to the liver. He said, 'If I were you I wouldn't worry about it, just get it checked out.' Fortunately, it was cysts that are not harmful, but when you are a cancer patient, news like this can be really scary, and he couldn't understand what my problem was. Even when I complained to his superiors, he refused to apologize. He hurt me badly."

30.
The Lists: Do's, Don'ts, Tools, and Treasures

WE LOVE LISTS, DON'T WE? Dave Letterman's Top 10 are certainly the best, but try these on to test your compassion quotient and help yourself and your friend or loved one with cancer live a better and maybe longer life!

20 more things people who have cancer want you to know

1. "I need to be touched." (Ask permission first, of course.)

2. "I want to be indulged. Even if I'm wrong, let me be right, just for now."

3. "I want you to help me believe in miracles."

4. "When you say you're going to do something for me, follow through quickly."

5. "Being sick is expensive; offer to treat me."

6. "Sometimes I'd rather hear about your day than share news about mine."

7. "You don't know how I feel. Please don't say you do."

8. "I don't want to hear that I'll be just fine."

9. "I don't want to be blamed for having cancer, *even if I may have done something to bring it about*."

10. "I may be extra sensitive to chaos and bad news. Keep it calm and positive."

11. "I am unique, so please don't compare me." Said one survivor, "Don't tell me how wonderful Lance Armstrong is, not letting cancer 'get him down' . . . you don't read about when he was down or puking or tired, and when you compare me to him or any other famous cancer survivor, I feel like I am less-than because chemo is kicking my butt."

12. "I don't like to hear how awful or thin I look."

13. "I don't like to be labeled as a hero. I'm just doing what I have to."

14. "I'm not contagious and feel horrible when I'm treated that way."

16. "I want and need privacy."

17. "It's hard to hear how scared you are for me. It's tough enough dealing with my own fears."

18. "I don't want to be looked at like a 'dead man walking,' even if I am."

19. "I need you to accept whatever I am feeling."

20. "The simplest gesture, like a text message every day or two, can mean the world to me."

24 fabulous things people did for or said to those who have had cancer

1. "I had two wonderful friends that came over to my house in the winter, days before I was scheduled for my mastectomy. They planted at least three hundred tulip bulbs in my front and back yard. I didn't make it back home until just a few weeks before the tulips bloomed. I will never forget the day that I saw those tulips bloom. I had finally gained the strength to come downstairs. It was breathtaking! Pink tulips filled our yard and they seemed to be saying, 'You made it! We represent the life that was given back to you!'"

2. "I asked my Facebook friends to inspire me by sending me something handwritten telling me what inspired them, made them laugh, or made their day. And forty people did.'

3. "I love to work with wood. When [spinal cord melanoma] paralyzed me, I knew I could not sit in front of the TV and rot away. My friends came over and lowered all my machines and put them on wheels so I could work again. Without this creative outlet, I would certainly go insane."

4. "I had surgery just before Thanksgiving and thought I wouldn't celebrate or miss the holiday. But one friend, unsolicited, sent over a HUGE tray of Thanksgiving leftovers. I felt both included back into the world and nourished."

5. "One of my friends bought me a special gift for every treatment; my husband also treated me to special things while I was going through chemo. My family had a 'Chemo Party' for each treatment, complete with snacks, beverages, and lots of prayers and love. It made the experience bearable."

6. "I live alone and had to take six months off of work for chemotherapy. My brothers paid some of my bills, bought me a month's worth of groceries, got food for my dogs. One even gave me a gift of $5,000 just so I wouldn't have to worry about expenses."

7. "While I was in the hospital for six months, a neighbor 'stole' my plant, took care of it, and silently returned it when I came home."

8. "My best gay boyfriend offered, without being asked, to sit with and care for my partner while I was in surgery and after. When horrifying complications suddenly sent me from dinner with my kids to flatlining and, twenty minutes later, into surgery, that same friend raced to my home to be with my kids."

9. "Two friends got together and brought over a cooler filled with tuna salad, egg salad, chicken salad, cut-up fruit, fresh berries, chunks of cheese, crackers, and nuts. I didn't ask for this; they just did it. It was such a relief to know that I had already prepared food just behind the refrigerator door."

10. "My sister Nancy upended her own life in California and came to Massachusetts to live with my boyfriend and me for a month after my surgery so that my boyfriend could go to work. She helped me shower, massaged my back every night at bedtime, cleaned our house. She never asked, 'What can I do?' She just did it. She left her own life behind to help save mine."

11. "My hairdresser would come to my home and do my hair and it really helped me to feel better when I looked better."

12. "I didn't tell anyone what I was going through—not my family, not most of my friends. My friend, Jessi, would ask me when my appointments at Sloan-Kettering were, and even if I told her not to come, she would simply show up in the lobby and sit with me. And afterward, she would take me out for a snack or lunch."

13. "A friend who had gone through breast cancer before me brought over her hats and other head coverings—let me know she had washed all of them and I could use them or not, whatever I wanted. No pressure. Bless her!"

14. "One person sent me a thoughtful card every week I was undergoing treatment. She never missed a week. I watched the mail for those cards. (Anyone can send one card.)"

15. "A friend, totally mainstream professional and conservative, showed up with pot/marijuana when my antinausea med repeatedly failed. It was hysterical to watch her try to roll a joint. I don't think she had ever rolled/smoked in her life."

16. "My friends did my laundry. At the time, I lived in an apartment and had to take my laundry out. Various friends would just come collect the laundry, during the really hard stretches, and do it, fold it, and put it away. HEAVEN!"

17. "One time I was camping with a girlfriend while I was getting chemo. She offered to rub my bald head. It was good strokes both physically and mentally."

18. "My girlfriends made it their mission every month during my treatment to schedule some kind of get-together, always with props, always

designed to make me laugh and have fun. To one party, they brought Groucho Marx glasses and noses that we all wore in the very swank W hotel. Making fools of ourselves in nice places became our MO. Just writing about it makes me cry—tears of joy and, of course, now tears from missing that cocoon they spun around me."

19. "My friends gave me a big care package before my surgery. It included an iPod with downloads they thought I'd like, decorated pillows and balloons for my hospital room, a designer hospital gown. . . . It was nice to feel loved and it was nice to have the most decorated room in the hospital!"

20. "My daughter's boyfriend's family, whom we had not even met at the time, created a beautiful tapestry, which had words of blessings woven into it. The intention of the words provided another visual meditation for me."

21. "A work colleague who had himself been through cancer brought me twelve big beautiful rocks to represent each of my chemo treatments. He put them in a large pile outside my front door. He told me to move one rock from the pile to the other side of the door so that I could 'see' my treatment progress. Each month I moved a rock and over the year the pile of completed treatments grew."

22. "The art office I worked in made me a huge sign with words of love and encouragement from all the professors, and they also made a jar with my name on it and collected almost a thousand dollars for me. It was nice to know I was missed and that people were thinking about me. Even professors I had never had classes with added their thoughts."

23. "As a teacher, I had less than ten days of sick leave left when I relapsed and needed chemotherapy. Colleagues from my school site and the district donated their own sick leave days to give me over one hundred sick leave days . . . (unused days at the end of the school year were returned to the donors). What a gift to know that I didn't have to worry financially about my bills!"

24. "I was a hospice coordinator of volunteers. Those volunteers got together and paid my insurance premium while I was on disability with NO insurance if they had not done this for me."

17 things people with cancer loved hearing

In the Help Me Live Survey, "I love you" is what people with cancer said they most wanted to hear. What follows are some individual comments that might give you ideas about words almost sure to soothe and support.

1. "I wanted to hear that people loved me; that they would be by my side through this entire ordeal; that they would do anything at all that I needed."

2. "I wanted to hear that it mattered that I was sick; that I made a difference in their lives.

3. "I liked, 'I'm going to the supermarket. Do you want to come with me, or can I pick up some items for you?'"

4. "I liked hearing, 'Can I drive you somewhere—to the dry cleaners, to rent a movie?' or 'Why don't I rent some comedies on DVD, and bring them over?'"

5. "During chemo, I LOVED: 'I'll think about you tomorrow at 10 a.m. when you get your treatment.'"

6. "Since day one I was told this by my best friend, and it helped me get through this: 'One day at a time.'"

7. "My husband said comforting things like 'It's so horrible what they're doing to you.'"

8. "I loved being told how much younger I looked. That told me I looked healthier."

9. "I liked, "It's normal to be terrified. It's okay to cry in front of me. I can take it.'"

10. "When people said that they probably had plenty of cancer cells roaming around their own body, and they might have some undetected tumors, too, it made me feel less alone."

11. "I loved it whenever someone left a voicemail and said, 'No need to call me back. Just thinking of you and sending love.'"

12. "Loved, 'It sounds like you're getting wonderful care from your doctor.'"

13. "'I'm so sorry you're going through cancer treatment' is wonderful when it's said openly with a kind smile and not a pitiful look."

14. "I liked, 'You look so good for what you are going through.'"

15. "Let's do something fun, if you're up to it!"

16. "Do you want to talk about it or are you all talked out?"

17. "What's your favorite soup? I'd like to make you some!"

20 great things to do for people with cancer (after asking permission, of course)

1. Research free services to organize help (such as Lotsa Helping Hands, Cleaning for a Reason, GiveForward).

2. Call or write, sending cards, letters, or even postcards. (Be sure to say you don't expect a response.)

3. Collect success stories about people with the same exact type and staging of cancer who fared well and ask if you can share them.

4. Visit—without expecting to be entertained.

5. Listen without interrupting, judging, or having to respond.

6. Treat them to lunch or tea.

7. Treat them to a massage.

8. Set up a prayer or silent unity group.

9. Bring pets to visit.

10. Do medical-related research.

11. Read to them.

12. Rub their feet.

13. Make a list of visitor rules for them to share with others.

14. Send a list of funny movies.

15. Buy a gift of special shampoo at a beauty salon.

16. Deliver meals (restaurant or homemade) or give food gift certificates.

17. Have their house cleaned, or clean it yourself.

18. Purchase gifts, such as easy-care plants that affirm or symbolize life.

19. Do their laundry or pick up dry cleaning.

20. Help their spouse, children, or other unpaid caregivers.

13 most outrageous things said to people with cancer

Warning: You may see yourself in one of these stories. Please, they are not meant to shame or scare anyone, but just serve as warnings.

1. "When I told a coworker the first time that I had a clean bill of health, she immediately said, 'But these things come right back, you know.' It was like she was disappointed that I was fine. She has no idea that I am clean and upright eighteen years later."

2. "I had a friend come over unexpectedly and got she mad at me (because I wasn't able to play hostess). She told another friend that I was rude and didn't keep her company or entertain her. I specifically stated that I didn't feel well and didn't want company that day."

3. "My mother, who had stage 1 uterine cancer, would say to me after I was diagnosed with stage 3c ovarian cancer that it was fortunate that they diagnosed her cancer early. It's not that I wasn't happy that my mother was okay, but I didn't feel like hearing that right after I was diagnosed with advanced cancer."

4. "When I told my office staff about having been diagnosed, someone mentioned recent articles about the correlation of stress and pressure with illness—therefore, of anyone in the office, she was not surprised that I was the one with cancer. It made me feel responsible for getting ill."

5. "One friend actually asked me out to lunch and proceeded to tell me that she was severing our friendship because I just wasn't 'fun' anymore. I walked out."

6. "One of the most incredible things I remember is how so many 'friends' let me go. One actually told me that she couldn't handle my

situation and that was that—she stopped speaking to me and doing things with me."

7. "'You should feel lucky that your husband hasn't left you—that happens sometimes' was said to me by a friend in the grocery store as a 'look on the bright side' kind of comment. I hadn't even considered that suddenly I was a liability and considered 'undesirable' as a partner."

8. "My mother had died just a few months prior to my own diagnosis. One person said, 'Well, you just went through this with your mom, so at least you know the drill.' All it did was remind me that cancer can kill."

9. "I had one friend say to me when we were playing golf not that long after my mastectomy (since reconstructed) that she thought I was swinging the club better because there were not restrictions under my arm for swinging purposes."

10. "I had osteosarcoma of the femur [and was in a wheelchair]. A woman saw me in the elevator at the hospital and said, 'Wow, I'd love to be pushed around all day—my feet hurt.' I'll never forget that insensitivity."

11. "[A coworker/friend whose father was in rehab said], 'It isn't as bad as other diseases such as alcoholism which affects the entire family more than just the person dealing with the disease.'"

12. "This person was sad to hear that I had leukemia, but knew I would do whatever to get sympathy and attention (laugh, laugh)."

13. "My spouse, who in all fairness was emotionally exhausted himself, asked me to stop 'milking' my cancer. We'd been married six weeks when I was diagnosed."

25 potentially dangerous (and common) words, phrases, and questions

You'll recognize many of the following from part I, accompanied by stories that illustrate why they're so potentially dangerous. But here they are in list form, for quick reference before you visit or talk with a friend or loved one with cancer.

1. "What's your prognosis?" (A medical term, prognosis is often associated with "poor.")

2. "Are you in remission?" (Wrote one survivor, "The term 'in remission' indicates that the cancer is lurking somewhere in your body, and it is just a matter of time as to when it will return.")

3. "How is your disease progressing?" ("Progressing" denotes worsening.)

4. "How arrrrre you?" (As Dr. Lawrence LeShan said, "If you treat me special because I have cancer, you keep reminding me I have cancer. Treat me like a human being.")

5. Or even, "How are you?" Cancer survivor, physician, and author Wendy Harpham wrote an essay about this in *Cure Magazine*. When she was first diagnosed, everyone asked how she was. "As if troops were gathering to wage battle against my fear and loneliness, 'How are you?' became a comforting code word for 'I'm on your side.' But within a few weeks, the chemotherapy began to take its toll, the shock and novelty of being a patient wore off, and I came to dread being asked, 'How are you?' . . . I found myself consoling those who asked, and then fighting the contagion of grief and fear.'"

6. "Are you cured?"

7. "When do you have to go to the doctor again?" (Let the survivor bring that up; she may not want to think about it now.)

8. "You should_____."

9. "You're so lucky." (Wrote one young woman, "Everyone told me that I was lucky because thyroid cancer is the best kind of cancer to get since it has such a high survival rate. It sucks to be diagnosed with cancer and have at least twenty people respond by telling you how lucky you are. I wanted to shout from the rooftops, 'Look at me, not at an article you read on the Internet. Ask me what my experience is like.'")

10. "I know a friend who went right on with everything she was doing and this was over in no time."

11. "You're so strong!" (Some like to be told how strong they are, but others don't. "I hated it when people told me I was tough," one survivor wrote. "I know who I am. But this was a battle I was not prepared for.")

12. "Are you a cancer victim?" ("Victim" implies helplessness.)

13. "I know how you feel." (Even if you've had cancer, you don't. As one survivor said, "Don't tell me you understand how I feel, because I don't even know how I feel, because this all happened so fast."

14. "Pray for a miracle!" (Although most people like to be prayed for, saying that they need a miracle implies a very poor prognosis.)

15. "You're going to be just fine." (As Dr. Lawrence LeShan said, "Don't tell me things you don't know anything about. Don't tell me I'm going to get better, don't tell me I'm going to get worse.")

16. Before chemo: "You'll have so much fun picking out wigs!" ("Fun" and "cancer" in the same sentence? No.)

17. "You even lost your eyebrows and eyelashes!" (Saying that can just make her more self-conscious.)

18. "You're on Taxol® (or any other drug)? That's bad stuff!" (Give hope, not fear.)

19. "Just be positive." (Sometimes it's not possible to remain optimistic. Better to encourage people to give themselves permission to feel whatever they feel.)

20. "I bet this has brought you and your family a lot closer." (If it hasn't, it can draw attention to the distance, and add to a patient's suffering.)

21. "Don't do that. It will wear you out." (Few people like to be told what to do, and most know how much exertion they can take. They don't want to be infantilized.)

22. "No one knows how long we have. I could walk in front of a bus and get killed tomorrow!"

23. "You just need to force yourself to sleep (or _____)."

24. "Don't get yourself all worked up." As Caring.com editor Melanie Haiken wrote, "Your loved one is scared, angry, or in tears, and you want him to feel better. But . . . a statement like this makes it sound as if you want him to put his feelings, which are natural and unavoidable, under wraps."

25. "Congratulations, you're all done (with surgery, chemo, or radiation)!" Someone said that to me after surgery and before I learned whether cancer cells were in my lymph nodes. And you never know you're all done.

3 subjects to avoid—or not bring up at all

As Rabbi Harold Kushner wrote in *When Bad Things Happen to Good People*, "Jealously is almost as inevitable a part of being hurt by life as are guilt and anger. How can the injured person not feel jealous of people who may not deserve better, but have received better?"

In addition, what may seem tremendously painful to the walking-well may pale in comparison to the patient's suffering. So when someone you know has cancer, especially if they're immobilized or financially stretched, be sensitive to possible jealousy or feelings of being marginalized or having their suffering minimized. Stay away from talking about the following:

1. Your upcoming or recent trip to Paris, Africa, the Napa Valley, or Saks

2. Your fabulous kitchen remodel

3. Your hangnail, which has been hurting like hell!

31.

How to Listen

LISTENING IS DEFINED BY *Merriam-Webster* as "a skill acquired by experience, study, or observation." But it's also an art, a thing of beauty that not only provides pleasure but also connects us to something much bigger than ourselves. As M. Scott Peck wrote in *The Road Less Traveled*, "True listening, total concentration on the other, is always a manifestation of love." And love never fails and always heals. To help someone without saying a thing, listen up:

- **Open your eyes.** Maintain eye contact, and don't give into the temptation to glance away at moving objects, especially when the speaker is talking about something important.

- **Move your body.** When you're truly engaged, your body reacts by leaning forward, and your pupils dilate. Though you can't control your pupils, you can move closer to the speaker. And if you're emotionally close, gently touch the speaker.

- **Keep your mouth closed.** When you're with a friend who needs to talk, remind yourself that you have two ears and one mouth and you should use them in that proportion.

- **Forget yourself.** It's natural to relate what someone else says to your own experience, but when you know someone really needs to feel heard, keep the focus on them. Don't worry about the wisdom you'd like to give. Simply listening reveals your wisdom more than anything.

- **Don't interrupt.** As tempting as it is to interject your thoughts, hold back. It's insulting to cut someone off when she's voicing an opinion, but it's even more hurtful and dismissive when she's sharing a feeling, especially a painful one.

- **Resist multitasking.** Most of us have become adept at cleaning off our desk or even checking Facebook while on the phone, but to really listen, let go of everything else. Even if you're just wiping the kitchen counter, it's easy to get lost in the sponge or the stain instead of your friend's story.

- **Limit distractions.** Turn off your cell phone when you're with a friend to signal that what he has to say is more important to you than anything else.

- **Be a mirror, not a window.** Listening is not about inviting people into your soul; it's about entering theirs. To let them know you have heard them, reflect back what you think they have just said.

- **Don't interrogate.** When you question someone too intensely, it can seem like you're more interested in learning something than actually hearing them. If you must ask questions, ask open-ended ones that give the speaker a choice, such as "Do you want to tell me more about that?"

- **Withhold judgment.** Quiet your inner judge and simply take in what the speaker is saying. Most people can tell when they're being judged, and clamp up accordingly.

- **Empathize.** In addition to withholding judgment, try to put yourself in your loved one's shoes. What is he feeling? How would you feel? This will help him open up to you.

- **Turn off your advice-o-matic.** If you're thinking about how to fix someone, you're not listening. If you must offer advice, ask permission first, and be willing to accept a "No, thanks."

32.
The Cheat Sheet

BEFORE CALLING OR VISITING a friend with cancer, remind yourself of some of the principles of respectful, caring, and compassionate communication. Remember:

- Keep it positive; don't bring up depressing or disturbing news.
- Come prepared with something your friend will be interested in discussing; think about their hobbies, interests.
- Offer to pay if you go out. Don't patronize, but show that you genuinely care and want to give them something.
- Don't ask too many questions about your friend's illness. Listen and take his lead.
- Take your leave early if your friend is tired. Ask. She may worry about hurting your feelings if she has to ask you to leave.

Instead of saying that, you might say this

If you remember the principles of respect, caring, and listening, helpful words will come easily, but sometimes it helps to have some alternative phrases at your fingertips, so I offer here some suggestions.

Instead of asking, "How's your health?" you might ask,

"How you doin' today?" If the answer is a tentative, "Uh, okay . . ." then you might follow up with, "I care about you and want to understand how you're feeling. If you don't want to talk now, no worries. But I am ready to listen when and if you do."

Instead of asking "How did it go at the doctor's today?" you might say,

> "So you went to the doctor today. If you want to talk about it, you know I want to listen."

Instead of asking, "Have you tried _____ treatment?" you might offer,

> "If you're interested in hearing about different treatments, let me know and I'll do some research for you."

Instead of asking, "Are you cured now?" try asserting,

> "You look terrific. I hope you feel great!"

Instead of saying, "I know how you feel," you could admit,

> "I'll never know exactly how you feel, but I'll do my best to understand if you want to talk about it."

Instead of saying, "At least they caught it early," practice saying,

> "I'm sorry you're having to go through this. I'm here for you."

Instead of saying, "Thank goodness your treatment is over and you can get back to normal," you might say,

> "If you feel like talking about it, I'd like to know how you're feeling now that you've completed treatment."

Instead of saying, "You need to think positively," reassure your friend with

> "It's normal and healthy to think negatively sometimes. There's even a book called *The Positive Power of Negative Thinking*!"

Instead of offering a cliché, like, "It's all for the best," why not say,

> "No one knows why such awful things happen to good people, why all of us have to suffer."

Instead of assuming that your loved one knows how much you love him, look him right in the eye and say,

> "I love you so much. You mean the world to me."

Instead of saying anything, hold a hand, touch an arm, or offer a hug.

33.

For Survivors:
Hoping and Coping in a
World of Uncertainty

MY SOLE PURPOSE in putting pen to paper to write this book—and it really did start with a pen and paper, when I scribbled the idea in my journal just a week after being diagnosed with cancer in 2002—was to spare survivors the added insult to injury that their friends, loved ones, colleagues and others may unintentionally inflict with thoughtless words.

But a funny thing happened once the book was released and, like a child, developed a life of its own separate from, though spawned, by me. Survivors themselves picked up the book. I can imagine them nodding their heads or laughing as they read about tales of sturdy and sensitive support or silly blurts or blunders. And I can imagine them crying as they read the true tales of abandonment or inaction tantamount to abandonment.

In revising and updating this book, I decided to include a section just for survivors, not so that we can commiserate, but so we can strengthen ourselves and revive hope when others dash, dent, or temporarily destroy it. Because, truly, that is usually the ultimate effect of gaffes: they diminish our hope for recovery, friendship, and love.

And, frankly, try as we might, we will never be able to cure foot-in-mouth disease unless we slap duct tape across the mouths of the entire population. And even then, we might see dreaded pity in their eyes or feel the sting of their avoidance. And, indeed, as we have seen, what stings one survivor may not faze another.

But, still, there is always hope.

And there will always be a well of sources, human and otherwise, waiting to be discovered! So what follows are some guidelines, in the form of an acronym difficult to forget, even for memories muddled by chemo or menopause. I call it "The HOPE CARD." Don't leave the doctor's office, or anywhere, without it. When somebody tells you their best friend or their uncle's nephew's sister-in-law died of your kind of cancer, or that you'd better stay away from that poison they want to treat you with or you just have to try that new shark gonad concoction proven (by whom?) to shrink tumors, or when you hear on the radio that a celebrity just died of the cancer you're trying to survive, remember that you do have control. Use one or all of the HOPE CARD cards to revive your hope and help it live.

H—Humor: Numerous studies show that humor and laughter build hope [see chapter 7]. Watch a comedy or children or puppies at play. Take a Laughter Yoga class. Hang out with your funniest friends.

O—Options: Psychologist Anthony Scioli said hope is rooted in empowerment and personal control. [See chapter 8.] If a doctor dashes your hope, get a second and third opinion. (Actually, I believe you should get additional opinions regardless.) Take control and know that there are almost always unexplored options. Create options for people who want to help you [see "R" next page], and know you have the option to assert yourself when someone says something you don't like [see "A" next page].

P—Protection (and People): When someone starts to spout a cancer horror story, interrupt with, "I like to hear positive stories." Protect yourself from negative people and news. Stop reading the paper; let your Debbie Downer friend's messages go to voicemail.

E—Empathy: Practice empathy for yourself and others. For yourself, realize it's okay to feel down, to think negatively, to get angry at friends, and to feel sad. To empathize with others, remember that most people blurt out of fear or ignorance; forgive them and you'll feel better. Seek empathy and social support from people who can provide it.

C—Connection: Social support has been found to increase hope and even longevity, according to many studies. Seek out whatever kind of support feels best to you, be it online or in-person support, activities with friends, church attendance, or whatever makes you feel a part of something, and good about yourself.

A—Assert yourself: When someone says, "But you look so good, you can't have cancer," come back with a funny, heartfelt, or simply honest statement like, "I may look good, but that's not how I feel." As one survey respondent said, "My older sister had seen several friends through fatal cancer illnesses. And I told her I didn't want to hear anything about their struggles or demise." This leads to the next point:

R—Request what you need: Let people know what words and actions will enable them to do what they want most—to help you. Make a list funny movies or books you'd like to receive. Write a letter or post something to your community asking for positive support. Ask them to refrain from telling horror stories or asking too many questions. And ask them not to disappear because they feel uncomfortable.

D—Deepen: Spirituality, prayer, and religion, which all involve faith and seeking deeper meaning, help keep hope alive. As psychologist Anthony Scioli said in *Hope in the Age of Anxiety*, a mission is a "particularly creative way to actualize hope" and to keep hope alive, you may want to "share your talent in the service of others while doing something, anything of enduring value." Participate in a fundraising walk or other event, if you are able. Volunteer to help someone else.

Afterword

"May you live all the days of your life."

—Jonathan Swift

June 6, 2011

IT WAS ALMOST NINE YEARS AGO to the day that I learned I had lung cancer, and began groping for a hand of hope to usher me through the dark theatre of the unknown.

Today I find myself in that theatre again. In three days, I undergo a biopsy to determine whether a nodule in my lung is malignant or just a piece of bodily flotsam and jetsam that mysteriously appeared in my lower right lobe.

When my doctor pointed out the whitish mass suspended in a sea of dark gray on my CT scan, a wave of fear engulfed me, carrying me back nine years. Then came the hypersensitivity and yearning for extra attention, compassion, and support. I received it from most everyone I told, but a few people seemed to minimize my fears, adding to my loneliness. Just like the first time, when I went through what I hoped was just a cancer scare.

But what differed this time was that, first, I knew how to ask for what I needed, and I mustered the strength to do so. Second, I knew how to better cope, relax, and nurture myself. And finally, I knew how to put myself in the shoes of friends and family who were frightened themselves about what might happen to me, or who just could not understand because they hadn't been through something like this, or who were so wrapped up in their own problems that they didn't see what to me was potentially life-threatening as significant.

In the grand scheme of things, a nodule of an undetermined nature is relatively insignificant. And certainly, compared to what others face, scanxiety is a pimple, certainly no tumor. Recently I talked with a friend, the mother of four sons, who was just diagnosed with breast cancer and will probably undergo a double mastectomy. And I'm worried about hearing the dreaded words, "It's cancer," that may never be spoken.

Fact is, no matter how ridiculous our worries may seem, sometimes we just can't keep them at bay, try as we might. This is especially true for individuals who have been traumatized, and as mentioned previously, one study showed that a quarter of cancer survivors had mental health scores suggestive of posttraumatic stress disorder.

This is why hope is necessary. Love is necessary. YOU are necessary. As Rachel Naomi Remen wrote in the foreword to *Help Me Live*, "This is not a book about cancer, it is a book about you. About the importance of your love."

Mostly, it is a book about hope. It is about the light, however dim, that leads us through the darkness; it is about the profound difference you can make by simply taking our hands and listening, because allowing us to vent makes room for hope to return. It is about letting it be not about you, but about us, just for now.

If you stumble, know that we will forgive you. We stumble, too. Everyone does.

And please know that because you have been here for us, we will remain more grateful to you than we can say. Hopefully, you will get back one thousandfold what you give, and your generosity of spirit will enrich you beyond measure.

As I sit with eyes shut, waiting in the theatre of the unknown, I realize that it matters not whether my nodule is cancer. I will deal with whatever comes. So I open my eyes and remind myself that I am here now, on our redwood-sheltered back porch, and I can see David's peaceful smile as he barbeques, and hear Brett's playful voice on speakerphone, and taste a sweet chunk of red pepper, and smell the Copper River salmon charring on the grill, and feel the smooth fur of Bean, Penny, and Jondo. All of this is real today.

I know that the light of love, hope, and faith that radiates from within and from everyone around me, will help me live all the days of my life.

And just one more thing . . . I promise!

June 22, 2011

You've heard of after parties and after-after parties? Well, here's my after-afterword!

I have cancer again.

Bleeping cancer.

#$!@$*% cancer.

If an obscenity comes to mind, please say it aloud. Just think what would happen if we all leaned out our windows and screamed, as TV exec Howard Beale demanded in the 1976 film, *Network*, "I'm as mad as hell, and I'm not going to take this [#$!@$*% cancer] anymore!"

So much for being in the moment. When it enlivens and evokes love, hope, or wonder, that's all good and well, but when you're in a pulmonary phone booth contraption, lips hugging rubber, following orders to *"Blow!!! Blow!!! Keep blowing!!! Blow harder!!! There's still air!!!"* until your chest aches, worrying that your lungs won't withstand another surgery, well, let's just say moment-to-moment awareness isn't always all it's cracked up to be. Even though I tried to imagine the chlorophyll green oxygen tank a few yards away as a helium balloon whose contents would allow me to shout, "#$!@$*% cancer" six octaves higher, I decidedly wanted to be anywhere else.

But you know what? I was right about what I said in the Afterword. With the support of family and friends, I AM dealing with it, the firestorm of feelings, the confusing treatment options, none of which will prevent new cancerous nodules from forming again. When one of my surgeons walked in after reviewing my nasty CT scan, he sighed, "It's the gift that keeps on giving!" (Still wondering what the return policy is. . .) And why do they keep changing the name of my cancer? Used to be "bronchioalveolor carcinoma (BAC)," but now it's "adenocarcinoma with bronchioalveolor features." What's next? *"Adenocarcinoma Featuring Bronchioalveolor, with Special Guest Star Remoflangiosis?"*

Hold on, though. Listen up! There are oodles of plusses to having cancer again, including that David is letting me be right 97.3 percent of the time, I'm not worrying about wrinkles, and we're getting lots of Tupperware from friends. (Okay, I'll give the containers back. . .)

Why would I point out the bright side of cancer? To remind you that I'm still living up to my name, but also to use what I have learned from thousands of survivors, including my late father (a misnomer: Dad was always early!), which is to lighten up.

Never forget that "I need to laugh—or just forget about cancer for a while" is the number one statement those of us who have been gut punched by this despicable disease want you to know.

So go to my website, www.lorihope.com, and check out the section that includes a dynamic array of videos, books, jokes, and other upbeat resources. Seek out what might help your loved one chuckle, escape for a while, or relax. Find a comedy, chick-flick, or action adventure film; a frolicking feline or canine; or a way to jump out of an airplane (with a parachute, please). Or send a meditation tape, poetry book, or spa certificate.

But first, consider whether distraction is desirable or even possible today. Sometimes things are so bad, there's just no escaping. That's when, more than anything, you might just say, "I love you."

⊒⊒⊒

Although this is the after-afterword, it's certainly not the last word. But I have to get back to work on my cancer treatment action plan. Before I sign off, though, this time for good, I promise, I want to thank you again. Dad used to say, "You can never be too rich or too thin" (actually, Dad, I disagree, sorry), but I do believe, and often say that you can never be too grateful. So:

Thank you for reading this.

Thank you for your compassion.

Thank you for helping me, and all of us slapped by #$!@$*% cancer, live.

Always hope,

Lori

Acknowledgments

ALBERT EINSTEIN WROTE, "There are only two ways to live your life. One is as though nothing is a miracle. The other is as though everything is a miracle." I look at life and the fact that I was able to write this book as miracles. But *Help Me Live* is not just a book; it's a project and mission and inspired by all those who helped me live to create it. I'm speaking not just of the health-care providers who helped me survive cancer, but more important, the family, friends, and others who nourished my spirit and soul through and beyond treatment.

There are too many people and too few pages here to thank everyone. Since the first edition of *Help Me Live* was published, hundreds more individuals warrant acknowledgment, including each person who answered my survey, helped distribute it, or granted me an interview; who joined and participated in my public online communities; who highlighted the issue of psychosocial cancer support in the news media; and who made this revised and expanded edition possible.

I hesitate to name any if I cannot name all, but some people must be recognized for breathing new life into this project. First, my outstanding editor, Veronica Randall, who made me stretch, breath, and laugh; Julie Bennett and Aaron Wehner, who supported a second edition and granted me extensions during my father's illness and in the aftermath of his death, as I found myself stuck in the inertia of grief. Thanks to the astute copyeditor Susan McCombs; and the original Ten Speed crew, especially publisher Kirsty Melville and art director Nancy Austin.

Special thanks to the insightful and intelligent Nicole Bazan, who Providence put in my path at precisely the right moment (at a Cancer as a Turning Point conference, no less), and eagerly offered her help; Judy Leonard, who helped make possible the space for me to write this edition; Mary Haake, who also helped create space for new possibilities; Barbara Cervantes Gautschi,

Michael Levine, and Alice Rose for adding wisdom, humor, and insight with their editing. Khelly Miller Agee, Roxanne Bruns, and Sandy Phillips Britt, who gifted me not only with their love but with powerful stories to share as part of their legacies; my mother, Ellen Crasilneck, who taught me that it was incontrovertibly wrong to be selfish and always right to be considerate and generous, and of course my father, Norman Crasilneck, whose support and encouragement motivated me to keep this project going.

My deep thanks to Kairol Rosenthal, Marc Silver, Mimi Avery, Shannon Kelley-Barry, and Ken Wilber, whose beautiful, rich, and informative essays and articles enrich the text immeasurably.

Gratitude as always to Brett, who is not only the best son imaginable, but also a dear friend, valued advisor, and editor.

And finally, my deepest thanks go to David, the most compassionate, generous, and patient husband and best friend on the planet, and an insightful editor and advisor, to boot. Without him, this book would not exist.

In addition, I must offer some apologies. Although I have changed most of the details of the stories and many of the names, you may see yourself in this book. If I discuss my own or someone else's smarting because of you, please know that everything is forgivable. This book is not meant to hurt, but to help and heal. It is written with love.

Once more, I offer a most profound gratitude to all of you who have helped me live.

Each one of you is a miracle.

Index